TABLE OF CONTENTS

1. ## INTRODUCTION
   - Note From Author — 1
   - Introduction — 1
   - The Importance of Food Safety — 2
   - Your Job is to Prevent Foodborne Illness — 2
   - Regulatory Agencies — 3
   - Management Responsibilities — 3

2. ## RISK FACTORS FOR FOODBORNE ILLNESS
   - Major Causes of Foodborne Illness — 7
   - Those Most at Risk — 8
   - Potentially Hazardous Foods (PHF) (TCS) — 8

3. ## TYPES OF HAZARDS
   - Bacteria — 10
   - Viruses — 14
   - Parasites — 15
   - Toxins — 16
   - Fungi: Molds, Yeasts — 17
   - Chemical & Physical Hazards — 18
   - Allergies — 19

4. ## PERSONAL HYGIENE
   - Employee Habits and Practices — 23
   - Preventing Contamination from Hands — 24
   - Proper Work Attire — 24
   - Handwashing — 24
   - Bare Hand Contact - Glove Use — 25
   - Illness Policy — 26
   - Hand Washing Poster — 27

5. ## FLOW OF FOOD
   - Controlling Cross Contamination — 29
   - Monitoring Temperatures — 30
   - Purchase and Receiving — 33
   - Storage — 34
   - Preparation — 36

Table of Contents

Cooking	38
Cooling	40
Reheating	41
Holding	42
Service and Display	43

6. Cleaning & Sanitizing

Cleaning Agents	47
Sanitizing Procedures	48
When to Clean	49
Warewashing Machines	49
Manual Warewashing	49
Master Cleaning Schedule	51

7. Pests

Identifying the Signs of Common Pests	53
Integrated Pest Management (IPM)	54
Deny Pest Entrance to Your Building	54
Prevent Access to Food, Water and Shelter	55
Hire a Professional Pest Control Operator (PCO)	55

8. Facilities & Equipment

Floors, Walls and Ceilings	57
Equipment & Utensils	58
Handwashing Stations	58
Water, Sewer and Plumbing	59
Refuse	60
Ventilation	60
Lighting	60
Facility Design / Plan Review	61
Maintenance	62

9. Active Managerial Control

Training	65
HACCP	66

Acronyms	71
Index	72

Chapter 1
Introduction

Chapter at a Glance

Note From Author	1
Introduction	1
The Importance of Food Safety	2
Your Job is to Prevent Foodborne Illness	2
Regulatory Agencies	3
Management Responsibilities	3
Quiz	5

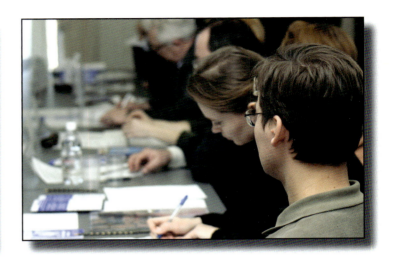

Note From Lisa Berger, Co-Author

I want to let you know that although I find humor in food safety, I take it very seriously and am very passionate about my work as a food safety consultant. Personally, I have experienced first hand the effects of a foodborne illness called campylobacter. I was sick for weeks and had abdominal pain so severe that I thought my appendix had burst. Professionally, I have been involved with many outbreaks of foodborne illness and in some cases, have worked with families of those who have lost loved ones to a foodborne illness. My goal in teaching these classes, writing this book, and working with hundreds of food service establishments over the years is to help reduce the number of cases of foodborne illness.

Introduction

You are most likely taking this class because you are required by your employer, prospective employer, or your health inspector to take a "Food Protection" certification class in order to get a job, remain employed, open an establishment, or to keep your establishment open if your health department has discovered you're not in compliance with food safety regulations. If you are like most people attending a food safety class, you are most likely dreading it. Perhaps food safety is not the most interesting topic, at least to your average person, so we will do our best to keep your interest while reading this book. We love to use examples of things we have seen and see everyday in food service establishments (both serious and comical) to illustrate points, and in some cases to simply entertain you so that you too can find the humor in food safety.

So, what is a foodborne illness? It is a disease caused by eating food (which includes beverages) that has something harmful in it. This something harmful could be a bacteria, virus, chemical, or physical object that could cause injury. Every year in this country, we have approximately 76 million people who develop a foodborne illness. Seventy Six Million! That's a lot. Of those 76 million people who get sick every year, there are approximately 325,000 hospitalizations and about 5,000 deaths. Yes, 5,000 people die each year of a foodborne illnesses in this country.

Let's compare this to another safety issue that we are all very aware of - fire. At a conference a couple of years ago, a fire marshal presented statistics on fire related injuries and deaths. He explained that every year in this country, there are approximately 3,600 deaths from home fires. (In 2006, there were a little over 2,500). These deaths were either caused by smoke inhalation or exposure to toxic gases. I remember sitting in my chair (thinking privately) – that's it? Yes, that sounds horrible on my part, but when you consider that we have fewer deaths every year from fires in this country than from foodborne illness and that we as a country are doing far less to prevent foodborne illness than fires, it doesn't seem right. We need to have the same commitment to food safety as we have to other hazards in our lives. You as a provider of food to large numbers of people (whether it be a hundred or a million people a year) have an obligation to serve these people safe food. Foodborne illness can be prevented.

This text book is based on 2009 FDA Food Code and will prepare you to take any one of the nationally accredited exams - ServSafe, the National Registry of Food Safety Professionals and Prometric (formerly known as Experior Assessments). Some of the regulations discussed in this book may be slightly different from the regulations in your state, county, city, town or jurisdiction as not all jurisdictions have adopted the FDA's Food Code.

The Importance of Food Safety

So, why is food safety important to you? Well, you don't want your customers getting sick from your food. This is the most important reason. However, there are other reasons that weigh heavily such as your bottom line. One illness or outbreak (which is defined as two or more cases) at your establishment could cost you tens of thousands or hundreds of thousands of dollars. This could happen as a result of an increase to your insurance premium, loss of business, damage to your reputation, the cost of correcting violations, and legal costs, just to mention a few.

Speaking of legal costs, what about the liability issues here? If someone gets sick eating food at your establishment, is out of work for days due to illness, or they die, you can and will be held legally liable. What if many people get sick? The liability issues grow exponentially. The fact is restaurants and handlers of food and food-related products have a legal responsibility to maintain a high level of product safety for their consumers. Many negligent companies have been tried in court and had to pay out huge sums of money as a result of these foodborne illnesses. Below are examples of a few cases.

- In 1993, $15.6 million was awarded in a case against Foodmaker, Inc. (who is the parent company of Jack in the Box), for an outbreak of E. coli. (A total of $100 million was Jack in the Box's total outlay for the outbreak).
- In 1996, $12 million was awarded to the families of children who were injured after consuming Odwalla apple juice.
- In 2001, $4.75 million was awarded on behalf of 11 children for an E. coli outbreak involving a school lunch program in Washington State.

In addition, you are required by law to serve safe food and it is your responsibility to be aware of what your local codes require. Many jurisdictions are now following the FDA model Food Code. Reading this book and taking a course is an excellent way to begin to understand your responsibilities for serving food safely.

Your Job is to Prevent Foodborne Illness

People are eating out today more than ever and it's up to you to provide them with the safest food possible. Maybe you're already doing a good job here, but my experience shows me there is always room for improvement. It's is funny to hear the comments from some of our clients - usually the ones who have been in trouble with the health department. "I don't know why we have to follow all these rules, you should see all the other restaurants nearby." Your job is to protect YOUR customers and YOUR business. And, what you see at these other places will come back to haunt them! These rules are not arbitrary, they are there to prevent foodborne illness.

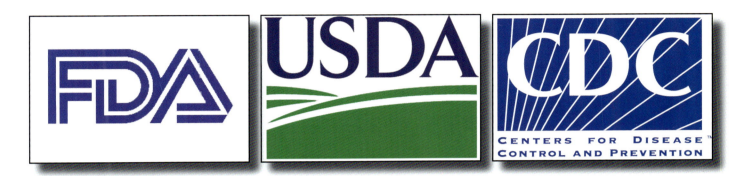

Regulatory Agencies That Will Help You Prevent Foodborne Illness

There are many regulatory agencies that are responsible for food safety in this country. For most of you, your business is most likely considered a food establishment. A food establishment is a restaurant, hotel, caterer, food service in a hospital or nursing home, a day care center that serves food, a mobile food establishment, or a temporary food establishment. In most states, regulations for food establishments are written at the state level. Most states have adopted some or all of the FDA (Food and Drug Administration) Food Code. For example Massachusetts has adopted about 97% of the FDA's 1999 Food Code and has additional supplemental regulations to those adopted from the FDA. It is up to the 351 cities and towns in Massachusetts to enforce this food code. Other states and local jurisdictions include all the latest regulations from the FDA.

The CDC (Centers for Disease Control and Prevention) is responsible at the national level for developing and applying disease prevention and control, and for developing environmental health, health promotion, and health education policies and activities designed to improve the health of the people in the United States. As far as food safety is concerned, the CDC is involved with numerous activities which include providing educational materials regarding food safety, investigating outbreaks of foodborne illness, and publishing weekly reports on various illnesses including those caused by food.

Finally, the USDA (United States Department of Agriculture) has many agencies, one of which is the Food Safety and Inspection Service (FSIS), responsible for ensuring that the nation's commercial supply of meat, poultry and egg products is safe, wholesome, and correctly labeled and packaged.

Management Responsibilities

If you are reading this book and attending a course, chances are that you are defined in the Food Code as the "Person In Charge" or PIC. It is important to know that the FDA defines "Person In Charge" to mean the individual present at a food establishment who is responsible for the operation at the time of inspection. Designation of a PIC during all hours of operations ensures the continuous presence of someone who is responsible for monitoring and managing all food establishment operations and who is authorized to take actions to ensure that the Food Code's objectives are fulfilled. A primary responsibility of the PIC is to make sure the code requirements are being followed.

Based on the risks that come with working with food, the PIC shall demonstrate to the regulatory authority knowledge of foodborne disease prevention, application of the Hazard Analysis and Critical Control Point Principles, and any requirements of the FDA Food Code. The ability to show thorough food safety knowledge is referred to as "Demonstration of Knowledge". The following is quoted directly from the 2009 FDA Food Code:

The PIC shall demonstrate this knowledge by:

(A) Complying with this Code by having no violations of critical items during the current inspection;

(B) Being a certified food protection manager who has shown proficiency of required information through passing a test that is part of an accredited program; or

(C) Responding correctly to the inspector's questions as they relate to the specific food operation. The areas of knowledge include:

(1) Describing the relationship between the prevention of foodborne disease and the personal hygiene of a food employee;

(2) Explaining the responsibility of the person in charge for preventing the transmission of foodborne disease by a food employee who has a disease or medical condition that may cause foodborne disease;

(3) Describing the symptoms associated with the diseases that are transmissible through food;

(4) Explaining the significance of the relationship between maintaining the time and temperature of Potentially Hazardous Food (Time/Temperature Control For Safety Food) and the prevention of foodborne illness;

(5) Explaining the hazards involved in the consumption of raw or under cooked meat, poultry, eggs, and fish;

(6) Stating the required FOOD temperatures and times for safe cooking of Potentially Hazardous Food (Time/Temperature Control For Safety Food) including meat, poultry, eggs, and fish;

(7) Stating the required temperatures and times for the safe refrigerated storage, hot holding, cooling, and reheating of Potentially Hazardous Food (Time/Temperature Control For Safety Food);

(8) Describing the relationship between the prevention of foodborne illness and the management and control of the following:

(a) Cross contamination,

(b) Hand contact with,

(c) Handwashing, and

(d) Maintaining the food establishment in a clean condition and in good repair;

(9) Describing foods identified as major food allergens and the symptoms that a major food allergen could cause in a sensitive individual who has an allergic reaction.

(10) Explaining the relationship between food safety and providing equipment that is:

(a) Sufficient in number and capacity, and

(b) Properly designed, constructed, located, installed, operated, maintained, and cleaned;

(11) Explaining correct procedures for cleaning and sanitizing utensils and food-contact surfaces of equipment;

(12) Identifying the source of water used and measures taken to ensure that it remains protected from contamination such as providing protection from backflow and precluding the creation of cross connections;

(13) Identifying poisonous or toxic materials in the food establishment and the procedures necessary to ensure that they are safely stored, dispensed, used, and disposed of according to law;

(14) Identifying Critical Control Points in the operation from purchasing through sale or service that when not controlled may contribute to the transmission of foodborne illness and explaining steps taken to ensure that the points are controlled in accordance with the requirements of this Code;

(15) Explaining the details of how the person in charge and food employees comply with the HACCP plan if a plan is required by the law, this Code, or an agreement between the regulatory authority and the food establishment;

(16) Explaining the responsibilities, rights, and authorities assigned by this Code to the:

    (a) Food employee,

    (b) Conditional employee,

    (c) Person in charge,

    (d) Regulatory authority; and

(17) Explaining how the Person in Charge, food employees, and conditional employees comply with reporting responsibilities and exclusion or restriction of food employees.

Not being able to demonstrate knowledge in any topic described above is considered a serious violation and may be grounds for revoking your permit to operate a food service establishment. So, study, study, study and enjoy the book!

Chapter 1 - Quiz

1. Many people attend Food Protection classes because:
    A. They are required by their employer to become knowledgeable in the prevention of foodborne illness.
    B. They are required by the local board of health.
    C. They have nothing better to do on their day off.
    D. Both A and B.

2. Consequences of a foodborne illness could include:
    A. Customers becoming violently ill and possibly dying.
    B. Lawsuits.
    C. Loss of business and harm to the establishment's reputation.
    D. All of the above.

3. The government agency responsible for writing the Food Code is:
    A. USDA (United States Department of Agriculture)
    B. FDA (Food and Drug Administration)
    C. CDC (Centers for Disease Control and Prevention)
    D. FSIS (Food Safety and Inspection Services)

4. One of the primary roles of the PIC (Person in Charge) is to:
    A. Ensure compliance with code requirements and other food safety regulations.
    B. Handle all customer complaints.
    C. Sign employee's paychecks.
    D. Hire all new employees.

Chapter 1 | Introduction | Page 6

5. All of the following are examples of "Demonstration of Knowledge" except:
   A. Understanding the relationship between time temperature control of PHF/TCS foods and foodborne illness.
   B. Being able to state required temperatures for holding, cooling, and re-heating of PHF/TCS foods.
   C. Being fluent in at least one other language than English.
   D. Being able to describe correct procedures for cleaning and sanitizing.

6. If an establishment does not have a designated PIC (Person in Charge) it could result in:
   A. A foodborne illness outbreak.
   B. High food costs.
   C. A citation or violation from the health department.
   D. Both A and C.

Answer Key
1. D 2. D 3. B 4. A 5. C 6. D

Chapter 2
Risk Factors for Foodborne Illness

Chapter at a Glance

Major Causes of Foodborne Illness	7
Those Most at Risk	8
Potentially Hazardous Foods (PHF) (TCS)	8
Quiz	9

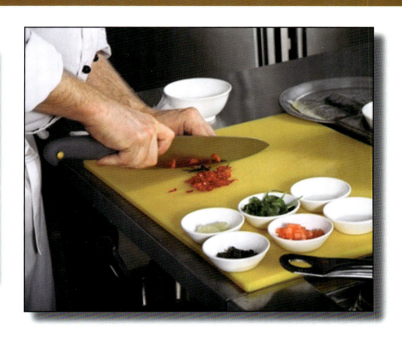

Major Causes of Foodborne Illness & How to Prevent Foodborne Illness

The major risk factors associated with foodborne illness can be broken down into several major categories: time and temperature abuse; poor personal hygiene; cross-contamination; and improper cleaning and sanitizing.

Examples of time and temperature abuse would include: not cooking foods thoroughly; not thawing properly; not reheating properly – basically not keeping hot food hot and cold food cold.

Examples of poor personal hygiene would include: not bathing on a daily basis; not washing hands regularly and thoroughly; not wearing gloves while handling ready to eat food; or not wearing a hair restraint.

Examples of cross contamination include: storing raw poultry or meat above ready-to-eat (RTE) food in a refrigerator or using a knife to cut raw poultry or meat and then using the same knife to cut cooked meat.

Finally, examples of improper cleaning and sanitizing would include: not removing all the food debris from plates before being sanitized; sanitizing concentrations not strong enough to properly sanitize; or rinsing utensils in a hand washing sink.

In addition to those categories described above, another cause of foodborne illness can occur from purchasing food from unapproved vendors. If you are required by your local food code to take this class, you are most likely classified as a retail food establishment. All retail food establishments are required to purchase their foods from reputable wholesale vendors who are in compliance with regulations. Here's an example of purchasing from a unreputable vendor: you have a friend whose mother decides to go into the pie business. This person decides that they are going to initially make all the pies in their home and sell the pies to restaurants. So, what's the problem here? Well, they may not understand proper food safety requirements or they do not have the proper resources to do so. Let's say this person also has a day care business in the home. You've got these pies being prepared and baked in a home where there are kids in diapers. Maybe they also use the kitchen counter as a table to change these diapers. The counter's not cleaned thoroughly – the same counter where the dough is going to be rolled. You get the point.

You should always be conscious of these major causes of foodborne illness whether you are at work or at home and during all aspects of food handling from the point that the food is delivered to the point where your customers are served.

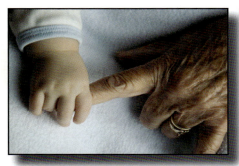 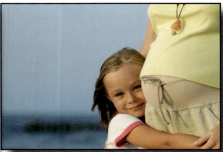 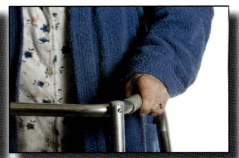

Those Most at Risk

Now that we have a general idea of what causes foodborne illness, lets talk about those who are most at risk for developing a foodborne illness. The most at risk include the very young, the elderly, those with a weakened immune system (these may be people who are on medications such as steroids or chemotherapy for cancer, they may have a weakened immune system because they have had a transplant, or they could have HIV or AIDS) and pregnant women. The food code refers to these groups of people as "highly susceptible populations".

These people are much more likely to develop a foodborne illness than the general population and once they do develop a foodborne illness, they are much more likely to suffer severe consequences, perhaps even death.

If you fall into one of these high risk categories, speak with your health care provider or research on-line how to prevent foodborne illness as there are unique food handling requirements for each condition.

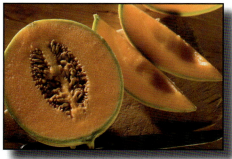 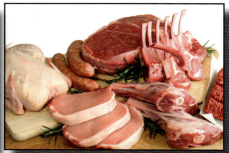 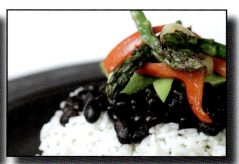

Potentially Hazardous Foods (PHF)
Time/Temperature Control for Safety Foods (TCS)

Just like there are some people who are more likely to develop a foodborne illness than others, there are some foods that are much more likely to make people sick than others. These are referred to as potentially hazardous foods (PHF) or time/temperature control for safety foods (TCS). These two terms are being used interchangeably in the industry so you must be familiar with both.

We like to categorize potentially hazardous foods (PHF)/time temperature control for safety foods (TCS) into several categories. One is high protein, animal based products like meat, poultry, dairy, fish, shellfish, and eggs.

Another category is "heat treated plant foods" which are basically cooked vegetables (and fruits) such as baked potatoes, cooked rice, baked beans, and steamed asparagus.

The third category we refer to as "other". Under "other", we have food items such as: cut melons, (watermelon, cantaloupe or honey dew melon); sliced tomatoes; raw sprouts (alfalfa sprouts, bean sprouts or radish sprouts); or soy products which include tofu and soy burgers; cut leafy greens such as lettuce and cabbage; and garlic-in-oil mixtures. All of these items are considered "potentially hazardous" and must be treated as such: they must be kept hot (135º F (57º C) or above) or cold (41º F (5º C) or lower). These foods sitting at room temperature can and will make people sick.

Chapter 2 - Quiz

1. All of the following are considered major causes of foodborne illness except:
    A. Cross-contamination.
    B. Poor Personal Hygiene.
    C. Purchasing food from Approved Sources.
    D. Time-Temperature Abuse.

2. An example of an unapproved vendor or unsafe source would be:
    A. Catching your own fish to serve in your establishment.
    B. Having someone prepare your desserts out of their home.
    C. Getting food from another restaurant.
    D. All of the above.

3. The following groups are considered Highly Susceptible Populations (HSP) except:
    A. Elderly.
    B. Young children.
    C. Pregnant women.
    D. College students.

4. Highly Susceptible Populations are at a higher risk of:
    A. Developing a food allergy.
    B. Suffering severe consequences from developing a foodborne illness, possibly including death.
    C. Becoming overweight.
    D. Both A and B.

5. Potentially Hazardous Foods/Time temperature Control For Safety Foods refer to foods that:
    A. Have been dropped on the floor.
    B. Are high in sodium.
    C. Are more likely to be implicated in foodborne illness outbreaks, especially if they are time-temperature abused.
    D. May have been treated with pesticides.

6. The following foods are all considered PHF/TCS:
    A. Shell eggs, poultry, garlic and oil mixtures.
    B. Cucumbers, canned sardines, coffee.
    C. Powdered milk, bread, canned tuna.
    D. Uncooked whole potatoes, garlic powder, cut pineapple.

Answer Key
1. C   2. D   3. D   4. B   5. C   6. A

Chapter 3
Types of Hazards

Chapter at a glance

Bacteria	10
Viruses	14
Parasites	15
Toxins	16
Funghi: Molds, Yeasts	17
Chemical & Physical Hazards	18
Allergies	19
Quiz	20

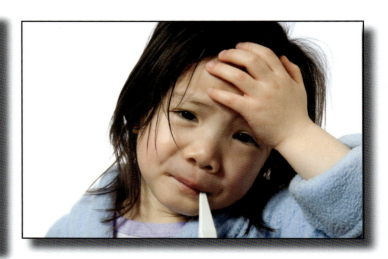

At this point you have learned about major causes of foodborne illness. We stress "causes" here because these are the things that we do or don't do that will make people sick. For example, the chef doesn't cook the chicken thoroughly (this is a time and temperature issue), the line cook doesn't wash her hands after taking a break (this is a personal hygiene issue), or an employee chops vegetables using that same cutting board that had just been used on raw chicken (this is an example of cross-contamination).

Now we will go into the actual things that we ingest that can make us sick which we call "hazards". There are three different hazard categories: biological hazards, chemical hazards and physical hazards. The most significant hazards to your food fall under biological hazards. Biological hazards can also be referred to as microbial contaminants, microorganisms or pathogens. There are six types of microorganisms that can contaminate our food: bacteria, viruses, parasites, toxins, yeasts and molds. The first four are considered pathogenic microorganisms meaning they can cause illness when ingested. Yeast and mold are called spoilage organisms and for the most part, these are not the microorganisms that make people sick. The four main pathogenic microorganisms that we are going to focus on are bacteria, viruses, parasites and toxins.

Up until very recently, bacteria was considered our greatest threat to food safety. Almost everything that we had done in our kitchens, whether at work or at home, was to prevent the spread and growth of bacteria. Now, viruses have risen to the greatest threat to food safety. In fact, of all foodborne illnesses, viruses represent 70% of all cases.

Bacteria

Although viruses are now our greatest threat to food safety, bacteria is also a very significant threat and the most difficult of all the microorganisms to understand. Bacteria are everywhere, they're on your potentially hazardous foods, your non-potentially hazardous foods, they're on your equipment, utensils, door handles, can openers, in your hair, on your hands, literally everywhere. In addition to bacteria being everywhere, it can grow rapidly under certain conditions. In order for bacteria to grow rapidly, there are six conditions that must be met and if you can memorize the acronym FAT TOM, you can remember these six conditions.

F = Food

"F" – "F" stands for food. Bacteria require food in order to grow and survive, just like other living organisms. The foods most likely to support the growth of bacteria would be potentially hazardous foods or time temperature control for safety foods.

A = Acidity

"A" – "A" stands for acidity. Bacteria require foods that are slightly acidic to neutral in their pH levels in order to grow and survive. If you look at the pH scale, you will notice that the scale goes from 0 to 14. Seven (7) is considered neutral meaning that it is neither acidic nor alkaline. Anything below 7 is considered acidic and anything above 7 is considered alkaline. Bacteria require foods that have pH levels between 4.6 and 7.5. Most all potentially hazardous foods have pH levels between 4.6 and 7.5.

T = Temperature

Very acidic food items, those below 4.6 on the pH scale, are considered too acidic for bacteria to grow. For example, vinegar, lemons, limes, and pineapples, as well as many others, are considered very acidic food items. Not only will bacteria not grow on these food items, but if, for example, you were to add vinegar or lemon juice to a potentially hazardous food, you would be adding a protective effect. The acid from the vinegar or lemon juice would not only help prevent some of the bacteria from growing, but will also kill some of the bacteria.

T = Time

Another acidic food item that most people don't consider "acidic" is mayonnaise. Mayonnaise is acidic – on a pH scale, it's around 4.2 - 4.5. Similar to adding vinegar or lemon juice to that tuna salad, that mayonnaise adds a slightly protective effect.

O = Oxygen

PH Scale

ACIDIC — ALKALINE

0 — 7 — 14

4.6 — 7.5

Bacteria Grows Easily

M = Moisture

"T" - Let's talk about temperature first. There is something called the "temperature danger zone" which is a temperature range in which bacteria will grow. Currently, the FDA defines the temperature danger zone as 41° F (5° C) to 135° F (57° C). However, the temperature danger zone may be different depending on where you're located.

Since you will be taking a Food Protection certification test based on the current food code, you must know the 41° F (5° C) to 135° F (57° C) temperature range. It is also important to know what your local jurisdiction recognizes as the danger zone because this will also influence hot holding requirements, in use storage utensil requirements, receiving of hot food requirements, cooking temperature requirements for fruits and vegetables that will be placed in hot holding, and cooking temperature requirements for products taken from a commercially processed, hermetically sealed container.

Now the reason this is called the temperature danger zone is because bacteria grows more quickly between the temperatures of 41º F (5º C) to 135º F (57º C). The longer your potentially hazardous foods remain in the temperature danger zone, the more the bacteria grows. The more the bacteria grows, the more likely this food will make someone sick.

"**T**"- This is where time comes in – the next big "T". To review, the longer the potentially hazardous foods sit in the danger zone, the more the bacteria grows and the more the bacteria grows, the more likely it will make someone sick. So, the maximum time potentially hazardous foods can remain in the danger zone is 4

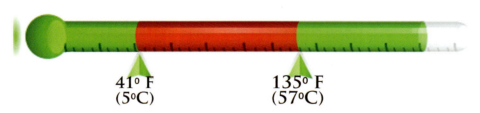

TEMPERATURE DANGER ZONE

41º F (5ºC)   135º F (57ºC)

hours. We in the food safety world call this the "4 Hour Rule". Potentially hazardous foods may remain in the temperature danger zone for up to four hours. Seems like a long time doesn't it? Well, it's really not. We're not saying that the product can sit out at room temperature for four hours EACH time we take it out of the refrigerator. We mean the time that it takes to receive and inspect the product, the time that it takes to get into cold storage, the time that it takes to prepare the food before the cooking process, etc. . . . When you add all this time up, it's really not much time. The "4 Hour Clock" starts over once a product has been cooked. Now keep in mind, you should never take something out of the refrigerator and leave it at room temperature for four hours

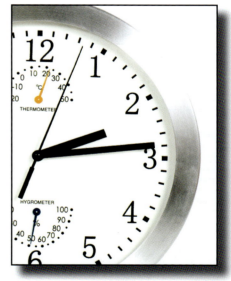

because chances are good that the product had already been in the temperature danger zone at some time. Also, some jurisdictions don't allow you to keep potentially hazardous foods in the temperature danger zone for more than one hour without getting a variance granted and submitting a full HACCP plan. (See chapter 9 Active Managerial Control).

"**O**" The "O" in our FAT TOM acronym stands for oxygen. Most bacteria require oxygen in order to grow and survive. There are other types of bacteria that not only survive in the absence of oxygen, but thrive and can produce deadly toxins. So, some bacteria need oxygen and some don't.

"**M**" - The next letter "M" stands for moisture. Bacteria need moisture to grow and to survive. Potentially hazardous foods provide the perfect amount of moisture for most all bacteria. In the food safety world, moisture is referred to as the water activity level. The water activity levels are based on a scale that ranges from 0 to 1. Most potentially hazards foods have very high water activity levels – from .98 to .99. The threshold is .85. Bacteria require foods that have a water activity level of .85 or higher. We can preserve food or change a food from being a potentially hazardous food to a non-potentially hazardous foods by adjusting the water activity level. For example, bacon has a very high water activity level, around .98 or .99. When we cook that bacon until it's crisp, the water activity level drops down to around .75 which will no longer support the growth of bacteria. That is why we can leave bacon that is cooked to a crisp at room temperature – it's no longer potentially hazardous.

You need to understand FAT TOM in order to understand how bacteria can grow and how it can be controlled in your business. You also need to keep in mind that FAT TOM only applies to bacteria – not any other microbiological hazards. Also know that although cooking foods thoroughly can kill bacteria, freezing will NOT kill bacteria. Although bacteria will not grow when frozen, it is still "living" and will begin to grow when the food is no longer frozen.

The following is a list of common foodborne bacterial illnesses. You must be familiar with the names of these illnesses, the foods most commonly associated with the bacteria and the most effective way to prevent these illnesses from occurring.

Bacteria That Cause Foodborne Illness

Organism	Common Name of Illness	Onset Time After Ingestion	Signs & Symptoms	Duration	Food Sources
Bacillus cereus	Bacillus cereus food poisoning (two types: emetic and diarrheal)	Emetic: .5 - 6 hours Diarrheal: 6-15 hours	Emetic: nausea and vomiting Diarrheal: abdominal cramps and watery diarrhea	Emetic: less than 24 hours Diarrheal: 24-48 hours	Emetic: starchy foods such as rice, potatoes and pasta. Diarrheal: meats, stews, gravies, vanilla sauce.
Prevention: Time/Temperature Control					
Campylobacter jejuni	Campylobacteriosis	2-5 days	Diarrhea, cramps, fever, and vomiting; diarrhea may be bloody	2-10 days	Raw and under cooked poultry, unpasteurized milk, contaminated water.
Prevention: Time/Temperature Control					
Clostridium perfringens	Clostridium perfringens or perfringens food poisonings	8-22 hours	Diarrhea, abdominal cramps and occasionally vomiting.	24 hours	Meats, meat products, and gravy.
Prevention: Time/Temperature Control					
Clostridium botulinum	Botulism	12-72 hours	Vomiting, diarrhea, blurred vision, double vision, difficulty in swallowing, muscle weakness. Can result in respiratory failure and death.	Variable	Improperly canned foods, especially home-canned vegetables, fermented fish, baked potatoes, garlic-in-oil mixtures.
Prevention: Time/Temperature Control					
E. coli O157:H7	Hemorrhagic colitis formerly known as E. coli	1-8 days	Severe (often bloody) diarrhea, abdominal pain and vomiting. Usually, little or no fever is present. More common in children 4 years or younger. Can lead to kidney failure.	5-10 days	Under cooked beef (especially hamburger), unpasteurized milk and juice, raw fruits and vegetables (e.g. sprouts), and contaminated water.
Prevention: Time/Temperature Control					
Listeria monocytogenes	Listeriosis	9-48 hours for gastrointestinal symptoms, 2-6 weeks for invasive disease	Fever, muscle aches, and nausea or diarrhea. Pregnant women may have mild flu-like illness, and infection can lead to premature delivery or stillbirth. The elderly or immunocompromised patients may develop bacteremia or meningitis.	Variable	Unpasteurized milk, soft cheeses made with unpasteurized milk, ready-to-eat deli meats. Listeria monocytogenes can grow at refrigerator temperatures.
Prevention: Time/Temperature Control					
Salmonella	Salmonellosis	6-48 hours	Diarrhea, fever, abdominal cramps, vomiting	4-7 days	Eggs, poultry, meat, unpasteurized milk or juice, cheese, contaminated raw fruits and vegetables
Prevention: Prevention of Cross-Contamination and Time/Temperature Control					

Bacteria That Cause Foodborne Illness (Cont'd)

Organism	Common Name of Illness	Onset Time After Ingestion	Signs & Symptoms	Duration	Food Sources
Shigella	Shigellosis	4-7 days	Abdominal cramps, fever, and diarrhea. Stools may contain blood and mucus.	24-48 hours	Raw produce, contaminated drinking water, uncooked foods and cooked foods that are not reheated after contact with an infected food handler such as salads and sandwiches.
Prevention: Good Personal Hygiene					
Staphylococcus aureus	Staphylococcal food poisoning or Staphylococcal Gastroenteritis	1-6 hours	Sudden onset of severe nausea and vomiting. Abdominal cramps. Diarrhea and fever may be present.	24-48 hours	Un-refrigerated or improperly refrigerated meats, potato and egg salads, cream pastries - particularly with food items prepared by food handlers with a cold or infected cuts.
Prevention: Good Personal Hygiene					
1. Vibrio parahaemolyticus and 2. Vibrio Vulnificus	Vibrio Gastroenteritis	1. 4-96 hours 2. 1-7 days	Watery (occasionally bloody) diarrhea, abdominal cramps, nausea, vomiting, fever, abdominal cramps, bleeding within the skin, ulcers requiring surgical removal. Can be fatal to persons with liver disease or weakened immune systems.	1. 2-5 days 2. 2-8 days	Under cooked or raw seafood, such as shellfish
Prevention: Purchase from Reputable Vendor					

Viruses

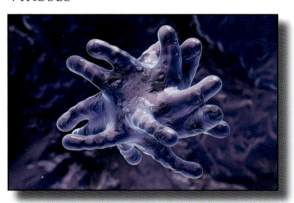

As indicated above, viruses are now the leading cause of all foodborne illnesses. Viruses are similar to bacteria in that they cannot be killed by freezing.

There are a couple of characteristics that distinguish viruses from bacteria. One, most viruses cannot be killed by normal cooking temperatures. And two, they do not grow and multiply on food like bacteria but require a "host" (a human or animal) in order to multiply. But, they survive easily outside of a host. Viruses can survive for weeks on most anything such as contaminated preparation tables, refrigerator door handles, utensils, cups, and plates or on or in any type of food or drink. And, not only do they survive, they are highly contagious. For some viral illnesses such as norovirus or hepatitis A, it takes a very small amount of viral particles to infect a person.

As mentioned above, most viruses cannot be killed by normal cooking temperatures. For items that receive no cooking, viruses can be a huge problem. For example, let's say an employee has hepatitis A. Chances are good that he or she has many of these viral particles all over his or her body and hands. If that person does not wash his or her hands thoroughly, and then cuts the vegetables for the salad without wearing gloves, the virus will get on the vegetables and make people sick. The best way to prevent viruses from getting into food is to make sure that employees practice good personal hygiene.

The following is a list of common foodborne viral illnesses, their names and the ways you can prevent the illnesses from occurring.

Viruses That Cause Foodborne Illness

Organism	Common Name of Illness	Onset Time After Ingestion	Signs & Symptoms	Duration	Food Sources
Hepatitis A	Hepatitis A	28 days average (15-50 days)	Diarrhea, dark urine, jaundice (yellowing of the eyes and skin), and flu-like symptoms, such as fever, headache, nausea, and abdominal pain.	Variable, 2 weeks – 3 months	Raw produce, contaminated drinking water, uncooked foods and cooked foods that are not re-heated after contact with an infected food handler (such as salads or sandwiches); and shellfish from contaminated waters.
Prevention: Good Personal Hygiene					
Noroviruses	Norovirus Gastroenterisis	12-48 hours	Nausea, vomiting, abdominal cramping, diarrhea, fever, headache. Diarrhea is more prevalent in adults, vomiting more common in children.	12-60 hours	Raw produce, contaminated drinking water, uncooked foods and cooked foods that are not re-heated after contact with an infected food handler (such as salads or sandwiches); and shellfish from contaminated waters.
Prevention: Good Personal Hygiene					

Parasites

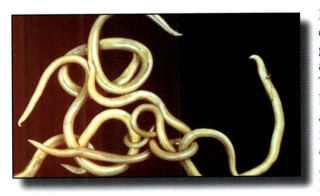

Parasites are very different from bacteria and viruses in a couple of ways. One, they can range in size from tiny, single-celled organisms to worms visible to the naked eye, and two, they can be killed by either cooking or freezing. They are similar to viruses in that they too require a host (a human or animal) in order to live and reproduce. Parasites are more and more frequently being identified as causes of foodborne illness in the United States. The illnesses they can cause range from mild discomfort to debilitating illness and possibly death. They may be transmitted from host to host through consumption of contaminated food and water, or by putting anything into your mouth that has touched the stool (feces) of an infected person or animal.

The following is a list of common parasites. You must be familiar with the names of these parasites, the foods associated with the parasite and the most effective way to prevent these illnesses from occurring.

Parasites That Cause Foodborne Illness

Organism	Common Name of Illness	Onset Time After Ingestion	Signs & Symptoms	Duration	Food Sources
Anisakis simplex	Anisakiasis	1-14 days	Diarrhea (usually watery), loss of appetite, substantial loss of weight, stomach cramps, nausea, vomiting, fatigue.	May be remitting and relapsing over weeks to months	Raw or under cooked infected marine fish
Prevention: Cook seafood thoroughly. Fish that is to be consumed raw must be frozen to -31°F (-35°C) degrees for a minimum of 15 hours or -4°F (-20°C) for 7 days.					
Giardia duodenalis	Giardiasis	7-14 days	Symptoms include watery diarrhea, stomach cramps, upset stomach, and slight fever. Some cases may be without symptoms.	Variable, 4-6 weeks	Water
Prevention: Wash hands with hot, soapy water before handling foods and eating, after using the toilet, diapering young children, and handling animals. Use pasteurized milk, juices, or cider. Wash and peel fruits and vegetables. Have well water tested annually.					
Cryptosporidium	Intestinal cryptosporidiosis	2-10 days	Diarrhea (usually watery), stomach cramps, upset stomach, slight fever.	May be remitting and relapsing over weeks to months	Uncooked food or food contaminated by an ill food handler after cooking, contaminated drinking water.
Prevention: Wash hands with hot, soapy water before handling foods and eating, after using the toilet, diapering young children, and handling animals. Use pasteurized milk, juices, or cider. Wash and peel fruits and vegetables. Have well water tested annually.					

Toxins

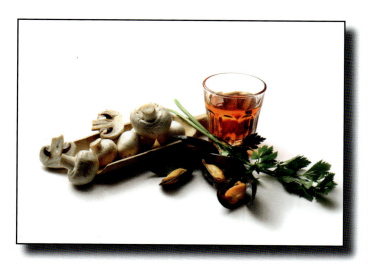

Toxins are poisons that can be produced by bacteria, carried by fish or shellfish, released by plants or are naturally occurring in some wild mushrooms. Bacteria can actually produce toxins as they multiply. As for mushrooms, people can become poisoned by these when hunters of wild mushrooms mistakenly consume or serve a toxic mushroom instead of a similarly-looking edible mushroom.

For the most part, toxins cannot be destroyed by cooking or freezing. The only way to eliminate a toxin would be to discard the food that is toxic. The problem here is that like other micro-organisms, they do not make the food look, taste, or smell any different. So, the question is how would we prevent these hazards? The most reliable way to prevent seafood and mushroom toxins is to purchase from reputable vendors. Toxins produced by bacteria can also be prevented by purchasing from reputable vendors, as well as by maintaining proper time and temperature requirements at your operation.

The following is a list of common toxins. You must be familiar with the names of these toxins, the foods associated with the toxin and the most effective way to prevent these illnesses from occurring.

Toxins That Cause Foodborne Illness

Organism	Common Name of Illness	Onset Time After Ingestion	Signs & Symptoms	Duration	Food Sources
Ciguatera Toxin	Ciguatera fish poisoning	1-14 days	Nausea, vomiting, and neurologic symptoms such as tingling fingers or toes. cold things feel hot and hot things feel cold. Ciguatera has no cure.	Symptoms usually go away in days or weeks but can last for months to years.	Humans become infected by eating infected marine fish such as barracuda, snapper and grouper.
Prevention: Purchase fish from reputable vendors.					
Scrombroid Toxin: (histamine)	Scombroid Poisoning	0 minutes to 2 hours	Skin flushing, throbbing headache, oral burning, abdominal cramps, nausea, diarrhea, palpitations, a sense of unease, and, rarely prostration or loss of vision.	1-2 days	It is most commonly reported with tuna, mahi-mahi, bonito, sardines, anchovies, and related species of fish that were inadequately refrigerated.
Prevention: Purchase fish from reputable vendors. Also, must maintain time temperature requirements.					
Brevetoxin	Neurotoxic Shellfish Poisoning	1-3 days	Numbness, tingling in the mouth, arms and legs, incoordination and stomach and bowel upset.	2 - 3 days	Oysters, clams, and mussels
Prevention: Purchase fish from reputable vendors.					
Domoic Acid	Amnesic Shellfish Poisoning	24 hours	GI distress. Sometimes dizziness, headache, disorientation and permanent short-term memory loss.	Infinitely for memory loss	Mussels
Prevention: Purchase fish from reputable vendors.					
Saxitoxin	Paralytic Shellfish Poisoning	15 minutes-10 hours Average 2 hours	Numbness or tingling of face, arms or legs followed by dizziness, nausea and difficulty controlling muscles.	2-3 days	Mussels, clams, scallops, oysters, lobsters and crabs.
Prevention: Purchase fish from reputable vendors. Also, must maintain time temperature requirements.					

Fungi

There are many different types of fungi, but those most common include mold and yeasts which are microscopic fungi that live on plant or animal matter. For the most part, fungi do not make people sick - they are considered spoilage organisms meaning they make the food spoil or "go bad".

Mold

Unlike bacteria that are one-celled, molds are made of many cells and can sometimes be seen with the naked eye. The mold spores give mold the greenish greyish color you see. Foods that are "moldy" may also have invisible bacteria growing along with the mold which is why food that has mold on it should be discarded. Some mold, however, is actually good and desirable in certain products. For example, certain types of cheese such as blue cheese and Brie have mold as a natural part of the cheese. Cheeses such as cheddar cheese or

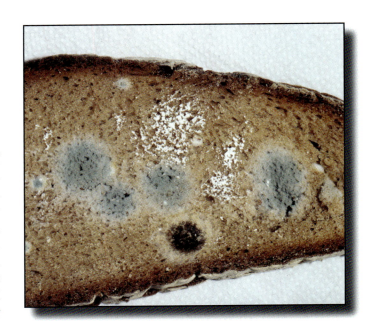

other hard cheeses should not have mold. If there is mold on these types of cheese, the cheese should either be discarded or, if possible, a one inch area should be cut around the mold.

Most mold is not dangerous, and only acts to spoil the food. Some mold can be dangerous and produce disease causing toxins in the food. Some people can also have allergic reactions when exposed to certain types of mold.

Yeasts

Yeasts are another fungi that spoil foods and beverages. Products commonly spoiled by yeasts include high sugar products such as fruit juices and concentrates, syrups, honey, jams and jellies. Like mold, if food has yeast growing on it, the food should be discarded.

Chemical hazards

Chemical hazards are chemicals that can get into food by improper storage of chemicals or chemical containers or by using chemicals improperly. These include any chemical that is routinely used in food service establishments: dish soap, hand soap, sanitizing agents, window cleaners, oven cleaners, or pesticides. There are also certain toxic metals which are classified as "chemical hazards" as well because they can leach into food if food is stored in these metal containers. Metals such as copper, lead (which is found in pewter pitchers), and zinc (which is often used for galvanized containers) are included as "chemical hazards" and have been found to cause foodborne illness and outbreaks.

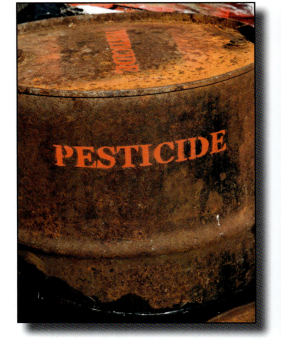

In order to prevent chemical contamination you must:

1. Follow the directions and safety precautions provided by the manufacturer of every chemical in your establishment.
2. Cover and protect all food when using any chemical, particularly pesticides.
3. Store chemicals away from all food and equipment.
4. Make sure all chemicals are labeled at all times. Never store food in old chemical containers or store chemicals in old food containers.
5. Make sure that pesticides are only applied by licensed professionals.
6. Never store or cook food in aluminum, copper, pewter or galvanized containers.
7. Make sure back flow devices are installed on all carbonated beverage machines.
8. Ensure any lubricants you use on your kitchen equipment are food grade.
9. Have the material safety data sheets (MSDS) for all chemicals.

Physical Hazards

Physical contamination happens when any object is found in food. This can be anything from a hair to band-aids to pieces of glass from a broken light bulb. Common physical hazards include: dirt, jewelry, writing utensils, wood, metal or paint chips, paper, packing supplies, plastics, dead insects, and rodent feces. In order to prevent physical contamination you must:

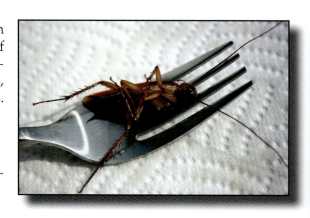

1. Inspect food on delivery for signs of contamination.
2. Store and cover food properly at all times.
3. Inspect all storage areas regularly for signs of pests or broken light bulbs.

4. Make sure that employees do not wear jewelry in food preparation areas.
5. Use hair restraints in all food preparation areas and in all food and equipment storage areas.
6. Avoid the use of loose pens, paper or other supplies in food preparation areas.

Food Allergies

Food allergies are becoming more and more widespread. Because of this, you must be aware of what the most common allergies are, what the symptoms of an allergic reaction would be, and how to protect your customers who have allergies. While more than 160 foods can cause allergic reactions in people with food allergies, 90 percent of all allergies are caused by:

1. Dairy
2. Eggs
3. Fish (e.g., bass, flounder, cod)
4. Crustacean shellfish (e.g. crab, lobster, shrimp)
5. Tree nuts (e.g., almonds, walnuts, pecans)
6. Peanuts
7. Wheat
8. Soy products

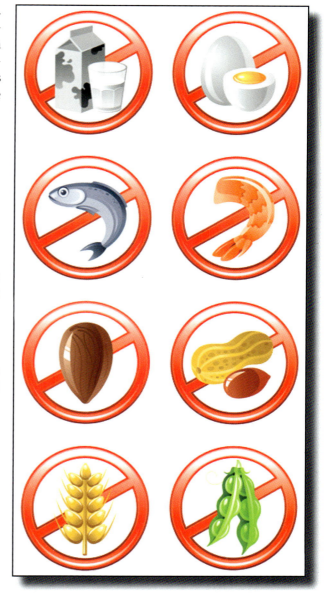

These eight foods, and any ingredient that contains protein derived from one or more of them, are designated as "major food allergens" by law.

Know the Symptoms

Symptoms of food allergies typically appear from within a few minutes to two hours after a person has eaten the food to which he or she is allergic. Allergic reactions can include:

- Hives
- Flushed skin or rash
- Tingling or itchy sensation in the mouth
- Face, tongue, or lip swelling
- Vomiting and/or diarrhea
- Abdominal cramps
- Coughing or wheezing
- Dizziness and/or light-headedness
- Swelling of the throat and vocal cords
- Difficulty breathing
- Loss of consciousness
- Anaphylaxis (airway constriction, skin and intestinal irritation, and altered heart rhythms. In severe cases, it can result in complete airway obstruction, shock, and death.)

Every year there are approximately 150-200 deaths from food allergies.

How to Protect Your Customers

The only way for someone to prevent an allergic reaction is to completely avoid the allergen. This becomes very challenging when someone eats out because they are no longer in full control of what they are eating. This is why it is important for you and your staff to fully understand the significance of allergies in your establishment. Everyone from the front of the house to the back of the house must be properly trained.

Managers and Employees

Managers or Owners:

If you are the manager or the owner of the business, you should have a written policy on how to deal with allergies. A great source for helping you develop a policy is The Food Allergy & Anaphylaxsis Network: (www.foodallergy.org). Your policy should address how the front and the back of the house will handle food that is prepared for a customer with an allergy. You must be aware of the menu items and whether or not they contain any of the 8 common allergens. It may be worthwhile to post a statement in your menu that says, "Before placing your order, please notify your server if anyone in your party has an allergy". There are certain foods that are more high risk than others for those with allergies. These would include fried foods, desserts, sauces, entrees with multiple ingredients or steps involved with preparation, and foods on buffet tables.

Front of the House Employees:

Any customer indicating that they have an allergy must be taken seriously as any exposure to the allergen could be life threatening. When a customer asks if a food they are ordering has an allergen, be honest. If you don't know, you must tell the person that you don't know. Ask the manager or chef for assistance. When a customer indicates that they have an allergy, this must be CLEARLY written on the ticket either by the server, manager or dedicated person. Once the order is taken, the manager, chef or other dedicated person should be responsible for the order. This will prevent the food from being contaminated in the kitchen and during service.

Back of the House Employees:

Before beginning preparation, make sure that all foods and ingredients to be used do not contain the allergen. Preparing food for the food allergic guest must be done separately from all other foods and on cleaned and sanitized equipment. You must avoid cross-contact. This can be done by: washing and drying hands and putting on non-latex gloves before handling any food for the guest; not using any shared equipment or preparation areas; and making sure that nothing spills into the food whether it is from splatter, steam, or foods being cooked or prepared nearby. Once the food is prepared, either you, the manager or dedicated person shall bring the plate to the customer. Do not place it on tray with any other food items as this may contaminate the order.

Chapter 3 - Quiz

1. Which of the following is not a hazard associated with foods:
    A. Biological
    B. Chemical
    C. Cross Contamination
    D. Physical

2. Bacteria require slightly acidic to neutral pH levels in order for bacteria to grow. What is the range:
    A. 4.0 – 6.5
    B. 4.6 – 7.5
    C. .75 – 1.0
    D. Bacteria will grow in all pH levels

3. All potentially hazardous foods (PHF's)/time temperature controlled for safety foods (TCF) must be held out of the danger zone. The temperature danger zone is:
   A. 41º F (5º C) to 135º F (57º C)
   B. 35º F (2º C) to 140º F (60º C)
   C. 40º F (4º C) to 140º F (60º C)
   D. 70º F (21º C) to 125º F (57º C)

4. Bacteria require the following in order to grow and to survive except:
   A. Food
   B. Moisture
   C. Time in the danger zone
   D. Oxygen

5. Freezing food can kill which of the following:
   A. Bacteria
   B. Toxins
   C. Viruses
   D. Parasites

6. Having employees practice good personal hygiene is your best defense in preventing which hazard:
   A. Viruses
   B. Toxins
   C. Bacteria
   D. Parasites

7. Edward has made chili that he is going to be serving tomorrow. He must cool the chili properly to prevent which illness:
   A. Salmonellosis
   B. Clostridium Perfringens
   C. Diabetes
   D. Vibrio Gastroenteritis

8. Cynthia had cut her finger with a knife a week ago that has now become infected. Today, she was making ham sandwiches without washing her hands or wearing gloves. Two hours after the sandwiches were served, several people complained of severe nausea and vomiting. The most likely cause of this illness is:
   A. Listeriosis
   B. Shigellosis
   C. Staphylococcal Gastroenteritis
   D. Celiac Disease

9. Jaundice is one of the classic symptoms of:
   A. Hepatitis A
   B. Salmonellosis
   C. Staphylococcal Gastroenteritis
   D. Norovirus

Chapter 3 | Hazards

10. Fish for sushi is most often served raw. The best way to prevent Anisakiasis when serving raw fish sushi is to:
    A. Cook the fish thoroughly before preparing.
    B. Add vinegar to the rice so that pH levels are below 4.6.
    C. Store the fish in the ice cream freezer.
    D. Buy from a reputable fish vendor who will have documentation that the fish has been frozen to -31º F for 15 hours.

11. As toxins cannot be destroyed by cooking or freezing, the only way to prevent this hazard is to:
    A. Never serve fish or shellfish.
    B. Make sure that all foods are purchased from reputable wholesale vendors.
    C. Boil all food that can potentially be contaminated with Ciguatera Toxin.
    D. Make sure that only the cook will forage for wild mushrooms.

12. The best way to prevent chemical hazards is to:
    A. Cook foods thoroughly.
    B. Never store food in old chemical containers.
    C. Make sure that all employees are washing their hands and putting on gloves before preparing foods.
    D. Purchasing foods from a reputable wholesale vendor.

13. All of the following are examples of physical hazards except:
    A. Grease that has spilled on the floor
    B. Staples
    C. Broken pieces of glass
    D. Hair

14. Which of the following lists encompasses all of the major allergens:
    A. Nuts, fish, soy products, wheat, and dairy
    B. Dairy, nuts, fish, eggs, tofu, wheat, shellfish, and chicken
    C. Orange juice, eggs, trout, shrimp, almonds, peanuts, bread, and tofu
    D. Eggs, peanuts, fish, shellfish, tree nuts, wheat, soy product, and dairy

Answer Key
1. C   2. B   3. A   4. D   5. D   6. A   7. B   8. C   9. A   10. D   11. B   12. B   13. A   14. D

Chapter 4
Personal Hygiene

Chapter at a Glance

Employee Habits and Practices	23
Preventing Contamination from Hands	24
Proper Work Attire	24
Handwashing	24
Bare Hand Contact - Glove Use	25
Illness Policy	26
Hand Washing Poster	27
Quiz	28

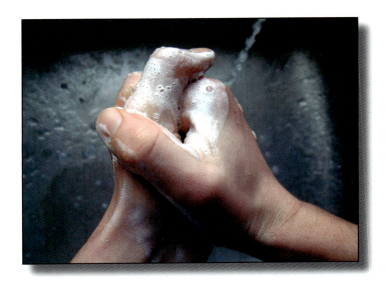

Proper personal hygiene is a critical component of your food safety program. Good personal hygiene practices can reduce or eliminate many of the contamination problems found in food service establishments. Remember, poor personal hygiene is one of the major contributors to foodborne illness and outbreaks.

We can break down components of a good personal hygiene program into three categories that focus on: employee habits and practices; preventing contamination of food from employees hands; and proper work attire.

Employee Habits and Practices

An obvious requirement when it comes to good personal hygiene is enforcing that employees bathe on a daily basis. In addition, employees must be in the habit of washing their hands regularly and thoroughly. While working with food, employees may not smoke, eat, drink, chew tobacco, or chew gum near food or equipment. If your jurisdiction allows employees to be drinking to stay hydrated, this may be allowed only if the beverage is stored in a cup with a lid and a straw and is stored to prevent the contamination of food and equipment. If employees cough or sneeze, it must be away from the food and equipment and guarded with hands or elbows.

There is also a way to safely taste food. This can be done placing a small amount of food into a separate container. Step away from exposed food and food contact surfaces. Use a clean and sanitized spoon to taste the food. Remove the used spoon to the dish washing area. Never reuse a spoon that has already been used for tasting. Wash hands immediately.

In addition, your job as the PIC is to make sure that employees' bad habits do not contaminate the food. Employees who play with their hair or touch their face, employees who put their gloved hands in their pockets and under their arms, or employees who sit on food preparation tables can easily contaminate food and equipment.

Preventing Contamination From Employees Hands

Employees must wash hands regularly and thoroughly. Specific procedures for washing hands are outlined below. Employees must keep fingernails clean, unpolished and short. They may never wear false fingernails or nail extensions, unless they are wearing gloves in good condition at all times. We recommend that you do not allow this as there have been numerous instances where false fingernails have been found in food.

If employees have open cuts or sores on their hands or wrists, they must wear a bandage and food service gloves or a finger cot. In some cases, employees should perform other non-food-related tasks until the wound heals. And finally, employees may not have bare hand contact with any ready-to-eat foods. This will also be discussed below.

Proper Work Attire

Employees must wear a proper uniform while working with food. Attire can be formal, as seen in restaurants where the chefs wear black pants and pristine white chefs jackets, or informal such as a company t-shirt or street clothing that is covered with an apron. You don't want to allow employees to come to work in their uniforms as they can and will become contaminated between home and work. If you do not have uniforms or a place where employees can change into them, an apron can be used over their clothing. Whatever the choice, employees must wear clean outer clothing while working with food.

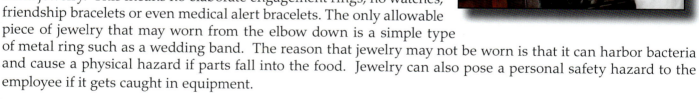

Employees must also have their hair restrained. A proper hair restraint could be a hat, a hair net, or some other device that will prevent hair from falling into the food. Keep in mind that what works for one person may not necessarily work for another employee. For example, a simple hair net would work well with an employee with short hair, however, an employee with longer hair may need to tie their hair back and then put on the hair net. Hair restraints are not required for counter staff who only serve beverages and wrapped packaged foods, hostesses, and wait staff if there is minimal risk of contaminating food and equipment.

Employees must avoid wearing jewelry, particularly arm, wrist, or hand jewelry. This means no elaborate engagement rings, no watches, friendship bracelets or even medical alert bracelets. The only allowable piece of jewelry that may worn from the elbow down is a simple type of metal ring such as a wedding band. The reason that jewelry may not be worn is that it can harbor bacteria and cause a physical hazard if parts fall into the food. Jewelry can also pose a personal safety hazard to the employee if it gets caught in equipment.

Handwashing

Employees must wash their hands and forearms for at least 20 seconds using the following procedure:
1. Moisten hands with hot water (sink must provide water at 100ºF (38ºC) or hotter) and apply hand soap.
2. Vigorously rub hands together scrubbing between your fingers, under your fingernails, your forearms, and the back of your hands. You must continue scrubbing for at least 10-15 seconds. It is the hand soap combined with the scrubbing action that removes the dirt and germs from your hands.
3. You must completely rinse your hands under warm running water and dry them with a disposable paper towel, heated air hand drying device or a room temperature high velocity device. Use

a paper towel to turn off a manual faucet or to touch the restroom door handle to avoid recontaminating your hands from these surfaces.

You must be aware of what your hands are touching at all times. You should recognize when your hands become contaminated and wash them to keep from passing the contamination on to the food you are preparing and serving.

You must wash your hands:
1. When you first arrive at work;
2. Prior to handling food, utensils, and single service articles;
3. Before putting on gloves to handle ready-to-eat foods and between glove changes;
4. Before and after handling or touching any raw foods such as raw meats, chicken, and eggs;
5. After using the restroom;
6. After touching any part of your body or uniform;
7. After handling dirty equipment, dishes or utensils;
8. After taking a break and;
9. After any other activity that may contaminate your hands such as washing dishes, sweeping the floor, taking out the trash, handling cash, eating or drinking, coughing, or sneezing.

You must wash your hands in an approved, designated hand sink that is not used for any other purpose. Sinks used to wash dishes or prepare food may not be used for hand washing. The hand washing sinks may not be used for any other purpose than hand washing.

Hand antiseptics or "hand sanitizers" may be used but only after your hands have been properly washed as described above. It is not a substitute for washing your hands. In addition, you may only use a hand sanitizer that is "generally recognized as safe" meaning that it is safe to use on hands that will be in contact with food.

Bare Hand Contact - Glove Use

Bare hand contact with ready-to-eat foods must be avoided at all times. This is one of the most important ways to prevent the transmission of viruses and bacteria. Single use gloves, deli tissues, serving utensils, and dispensing equipment can eliminate the bare hand contact for all ready-to-eat foods. Ready-to-eat foods include sandwiches, salads, cookies, ice, bread, pizza, garnish - basically, any food that requires no cooking or further cooking or washing before being consumed.

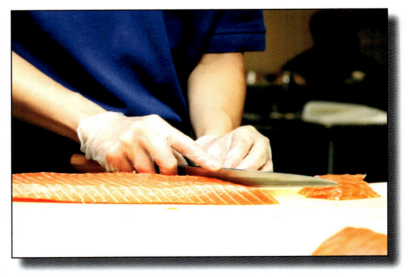

As for gloves, they come in various sizes and materials to fit the tasks and individuals who use them. Use loose, easy to change gloves when you are changing tasks often, form fitting gloves for longer periods of performing the same task, and only non-latex gloves, particularly for those who are allergic to latex. Some jurisdictions prohibit the use of latex gloves altogether as this could be an issue for customers with latex allergies. It is important for the manager to provide the right glove for the right job, this encourages proper use.

Gloves are never a replacement for hand washing; they are used in addition to hand washing. You must wash and dry your hands thoroughly before you put on a fresh pair of gloves. Gloves can only be used for one task such as working with ready-to-eat food or raw food and then must be discarded when damaged, soiled or when interruptions occur.

Make sure you wash your hands and change your gloves after any activity that may have contaminated your gloved hands such as coughing or sneezing, touching any part of your body or uniform, after handling dirty equipment, dishes or utensils, and whenever you change tasks.

Illness Policy

All personal hygiene programs must include an illness policy. An illness policy is your establishments' policy on how to handle employees who either have symptoms of a foodborne illness or have been diagnosed with a foodborne illness. It is required that you maintain an illness policy that outlines the actions taken based on any symptoms, diseases and/or health status of your employees and that requires employees to report illnesses promptly. Below is a chart that you can use when you begin developing your own policy. Most health departments will also be able to provide you with a sample policy that is more specific to local regulations. As the manager or Person-In-Charge (PIC), you have responsibilities for implementing and maintaining this illness policy, including:

1. "Restricting" or "excluding" employees from working depending on the symptoms/diseases an employee is exhibiting. It is important to understand the difference between the two of these. To "restrict" means to limit the activities of a food employee so that there is no risk of spreading the disease through food. Employees that are restricted can not handle exposed food, clean equipment, utensils, linens or unwrapped single-service/single-use articles. To "exclude" means to prevent a person from working as an employee in a food establishment or entering a food establishment as an employee. Employees shouldn't come in to visit or even pick up a paycheck when they are excluded.
2. Reviewing the illness policy with all employees and making sure that this is reviewed on a regular basis - at least annually. It's also a good idea to post this illness policy on an employee bulletin board so it is easily accessed by all employees if questions arise.
3. Making sure that all new employees are trained in the illness policy before they begin work.
4. In addition, it's a good idea to give two copies of the illness policy to all employees. One copy is for them to sign and keep on file with employee or other food safety records and the other is for them to take home. It is important that the manger or (PIC) is approachable so there is no fear of reporting illness that can affect the safety of the food you are serving.

IF	THEN
Employee has a fever or sore throat with fever.	Restrict the employee from working with or around food or exclude the employee from work if you serve a high-risk population.
Employee has an infected cut or an infected open sore.	Restrict the employee from working with or around food.
Employee has one or both: vomiting or diarrhea	Exclude the employee from the establishment until they are symptom free for 24 hours or they have a note from a medical provider.
Employee has jaundice.	Exclude for at least 7 days from onset, notify your local health department. Return to work only after approval from health department.
Employee has been diagnosed with a foodborne illness: Salmonella Typhi, Shigella spp., Shiga toxin-producing Escherichia coli and other Enterohemorrhagic Escherichia coli, Hepatitis A, or Norovirus.	Exclude the employee from the establishment and notify your local health department. May return to work only after approval from health department.
Employee lives with someone diagnosed with Hepatitis A or Salmonella typhi.	Exclude the employee from work and notify the local health department. May return to work only after approval from health department.

Chapter 4 - Extras

EFFECTIVE HANDWASHING
7 Steps to Prevent the Spread of Germs

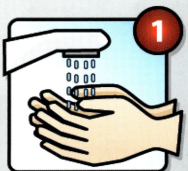

1. Turn on water to a comfortable temperature and moisten hands and wrists.

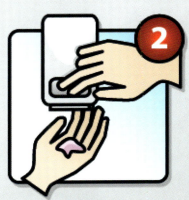

2. Apply a generous portion of liquid soap.

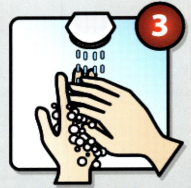

3. Generate a heavy lather and wash well for approx. 15 seconds. Clean between fingers, nail beds, under fingernails and backs of hands

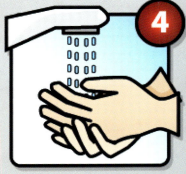

4. Rinse well under running water, keeping hands low in sink to prevent splashing.

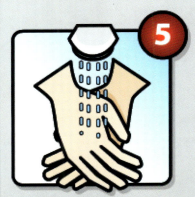

5. Hold hands so that water flows from the wrist to fingertips.

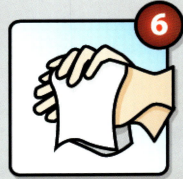

6. Dry hands completely with clean paper towels.

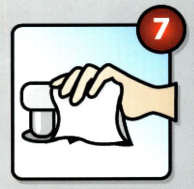

7. Use the paper towel to turn off the faucet so your hands remain clean.

Chapter 4 - Quiz

1. All of the following are bad personal habits that could contaminate the food except:
    A. Employees that touch their hair often.
    B. Employees that pick their teeth.
    C. Employees that are rude.
    D. Employees that put their hand in their pockets and under their arms.

2. Food could be easily contaminated by an employee who:
    A. Has several tattoos.
    B. Has their nose pierced.
    C. Wears shorts and open toed shoes to work.
    D. Has several rings and bracelets on each hand.

3. Drinking in the kitchen or other food preparation area is:
    A. Never allowed.
    B. Allowed only if the beverage is in a covered container and stored away from food and equipment.
    C. Allowed only if it does not contain alcohol.
    D. Allowed if it is done out of the view of customers.

4. Hands must be washed after which of the following tasks:
    A. Between handling raw food and cooked or RTE food.
    B. After coughing or sneezing.
    C. After using the restroom.
    D. All of the above.

5. The primary purpose of gloves is to:
    A. Keep employees hands clean and dry.
    B. Keep employees hands warm when working with frozen food.
    C. Save time- employees do not have to wash their hands as often when they are wearing gloves.
    D. Prevent bare hand contact with RTE food.

6. When washing hands employees must:
    A. Use soap, hot water (at least 100 degrees) and scrub for 10-15 seconds.
    B. Use soap, cold water (70 degrees or colder) and scrub for 10-15 seconds.
    C. Wear gloves.
    D. Use hand sanitizer instead of soap.

7. If an employee is experiencing symptoms of foodborne illness such as vomiting or diarrhea they must:
    A. Go to doctor immediately.
    B. Notify the PIC and stay home until they have been symptom free for at least 24 hours.
    C. Take medicine to control the symptoms during their shift.
    D. Be restricted to washing dishes, cleaning or working at the cash register.

8. An employee that has been diagnosed with_____ must be excluded from the operation and the health department must be notified:
    A. A food allergy
    B. Hepatitis C
    C. Hepatitis A
    D. AIDS/HIV

Answer Key
1. C   2. D   3. B   4. D   5. D   6. A   7. B   8. C

Chapter 5
Flow of Food

Chapter at a Glance

Controlling Cross Contamination	29
Monitoring Temperatures	30
Purchase and Receiving	33
Storage	34
Preparation	36
Cooking	38
Cooling	40
Reheating	41
Holding	42
Service and Display	43
Quiz	44

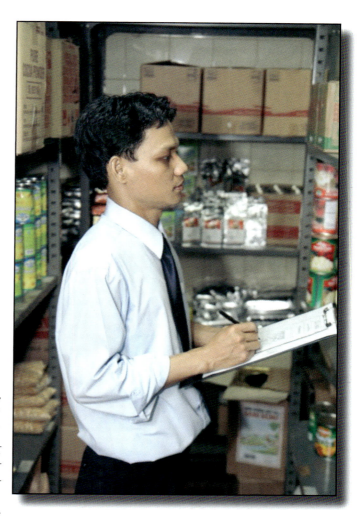

When it comes to food safety, there are common themes at each step in the flow of food from purchasing to serving. These include preventing cross contamination, maintaining time and temperature control, and assuring that employees are practicing good personal hygiene at all times. We've already discussed personal hygiene issues in Chapter 4, so we will begin focusing here on controlling cross contamination and proper ways for monitoring temperatures. Then, we will discuss proper ways to handle food during each step in the flow of food from: purchasing and receiving; storing food and equipment; preparing; cooking; cooling; reheating; holding; and serving or displaying the food.

Controlling Cross Contamination

As discussed in previous sections, cross contamination is one of the major causes of foodborne illnesses and can easily occur during preparation. This happens when bacteria or other pathogens are transferred from one food or item to another. For example, if an employee cuts raw chicken on a cutting board and then immediately begins cutting lettuce for a salad on that same board, the bacteria from the raw chicken will now be on the lettuce. The challenge here is that if you did not witness this, it's not obvious that cross contamination has occurred because you cannot see the bacteria.

One of the best ways to prevent this type of cross contamination is to assign specific equipment for specific food items. A great example of this, and something that has become very popular, is using color coded cutting boards. For example, yellow is most often used for raw poultry and green for produce. Although you may not be able to see the bacteria on the lettuce, if you see someone using a yellow cutting board for the lettuce, it is almost as if you can see cross contamination occurring. In addition to being used for cutting boards, this color-coding system is used for all types of equipment such as tongs, knives, spatulas, scoops, pan covers, and even thermometers.

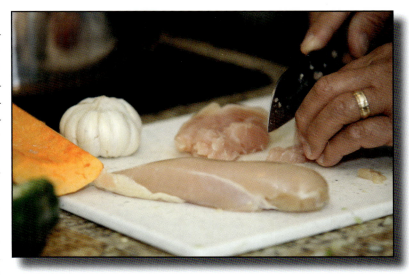

Another great way to prevent cross contamination is by preparing raw foods in a separate location from cooked or ready-to-eat (RTE) foods. Larger restaurants and food service institutions often have refrigerators or cold preparation rooms designated just for the preparation of raw meat, fish, or poultry. The majority of food establishments are limited in space and they do not have this capability. In this case, a great way to prevent cross contamination is by preparing raw food at a separate time than RTE foods.

Cross contamination can also be prevented by making sure that all equipment, work surfaces and utensils have been cleaned and sanitized before use or when changing tasks. For example, after cutting raw chicken, the cutting board, the knife and the preparation table must be cleaned and sanitized before cutting raw fish.

The last two significant ways to prevent cross contamination are to wash your hands and change your gloves when changing tasks, and to wash your hands and change your gloves before you change tasks. (Oh, did I say that twice?)

Monitoring Temperatures

As temperatures of potentially hazardous foods (PHF's)/time temperature controlled for safety foods (TCS) must be monitored during most steps in the flow of food, let's talk about thermometers – when to use them, how to use them, and the various types of thermometers.

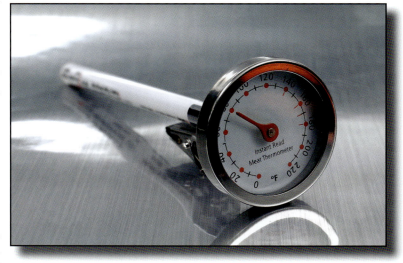

First, you must check product temperatures during receiving as you must be assured that all PHF's/ TCS food being delivered are 41º F (5º C) or below (shellfish and eggs are the exception as these may be received at 45º F (7º C) or colder – see specific requirements below). For delivery of hot foods, they must be received at 135º F (57º C) or higher.

Then, you will be monitoring temperatures during preparation – particularly if you will be preparing large quantities of PHF's/TCS foods. You must be monitoring your cooking temperatures to assure that harmful pathogens are reduced to safe numbers. Food in hot or cold holding will need to be monitored to assure that they remain out of the temperature danger zone. Temperatures must be monitored during cooling to make sure that time and temperature parameters are being met. Temperatures must be monitored when reheating food that will be going into hot holding. And finally, temperatures must be monitored during service of potentially hazardous food on display such as a buffet.

For meat, fish, or poultry, you should submerge the thermometer in the thickest part. For packaged foods such as vacuum packaged meats, you can put the thermometer between two packages.

For other packaged foods such as milk or prepared salads in containers, you can open the container and check the internal temperature of the food. For soups, stocks or stews, you should submerge the thermometer in the center of the product. Make sure that your thermometer does not touch the bottom or the sides of the container.

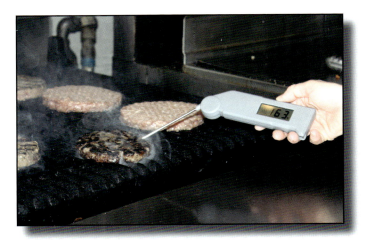
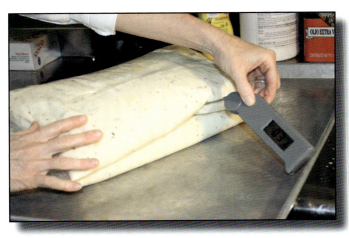

Keep in mind that your thermometer is considered a food contact surface and must be cleaned and sanitized before and after using it. It also must be cleaned and sanitized each time you change from one food item to another. And finally, you should never put a dirty thermometer back into it's case.

Thermometers

Thermometer photos courtesy of Thermoworks.com

Common Name	Considerations	Speed	Suggested Use
Laser Infrared	Measures surface temperature only. Does not touch food so it does not need to be sanitized between uses. Minimizes the risk of cross contamination. Cannot be used through glass or any other packaging. Must be calibrated by manufacturer.	Instant	This thermometer should be used as more of a screening device as it measures surface temperatures only. Works better on hot food stirred thoroughly versus cold foods. For record keeping or documentation, internal temperatures are required using probe type thermometers described below.
Bimetal (oven-safe) Thermometer	This thermometer can be placed in food while cooking. It cannot measure thin food. It cannot be calibrated and the risk of this breaking in food should limit it's use. Also, the heat conduction of metal shield can cause false high reading.	1-2 minutes	Placement: 2 inches deep in thickest part of food. Suggested Use: roasts, casseroles, and soups.

Common Name	Considerations	Speed	Suggested Use
Bimetal Stem Food Thermometer	This cannot be placed in food while cooking - it can be used for foods that have just been cooked or foods in hot or cold holding. It is easily calibrated with a wrench or thermometer case. This thermometer must be inserted 2-3 inches in the food for an accurate reading. Does not work well with thin foods.	15-30 seconds	Placement: 2 to 2-1/2 inches deep in thickest part of food. Suggested Use: roasts, casseroles, soups, stews, and protein salads such as chicken or tuna salads.
Thermocouple / Thermopen	Digital for easy reading. Can be used for various food types - liquids, solids, thick or thin. This is my favorite and most versatile thermometer. It can be calibrated, however, does not calibrate as easily as bimetal stem food thermometer.	3-5 seconds	Placement: 1/4 inch deep or deeper. Suggested Use: most everything. Particularly useful for hamburger patties, pork chops, thin fish or chicken.
Thermocouple / Thermistor	Digital for easy reading. Has numerous attachments: 1. Immersion probe for liquids; 2. Penetration probes for thin items (burgers, chicken breast, pork chops); 3. Surface probes for surface temperatures of grills; 4. Air probes to measure air temperature in refrigerators, freezers and dry storage areas.	Instant to 10 seconds	Placement and suggested Use: Depends on probe.
Time/Temperature Indicator (TTI)	A TTI is not considered a "thermometer", however, can be used to determine if products have been cooked to minimal internal temperatures.	5-10 seconds	Follow manufacturers instructions on placement. Suggested Use: to determine cooking temperatures for hamburgers or chicken.

Calibrating your thermometer

Occasionally, thermometers will need to be calibrated to make sure they are accurate. This should be done for all new thermometers, those that may have been dropped, or those you suspect are not accurate. Many thermometers may be calibrated by hand, others need to be returned to the manufacturer.

The best way to calibrate a thermometer is by using the "ice point method". To do this, fill a container with ice then fill the air gaps with water. Then, submerge the thermometer sensor in this ice water and let it sit for 30-60 seconds. You may want to stir the ice water to assure even temperature. This ice water will always be 32ºF (0ºC). If the thermometer does not read 32ºF (0ºC), the thermometer should be adjusted according to the manufacturers directions. On a bimetallic stem thermometer, this is usually done by holding the adjusting nut below the dial with a wrench while spinning the dial to read 32ºF (0ºC). Some more sophisticated thermometers have a reset button that will set the temperature to 32ºF (0ºC).

You can also use the "boiling point method". To do this, place thermometer sensor in boiling water. At sea level, water will boil at exactly 212ºF (100ºC). If the thermometer does not read 212ºF (100ºC), it should be adjusted the same way as described above.

The preferred method for calibrating a thermometer is by using the ice point method since boiling points vary at different altitudes.

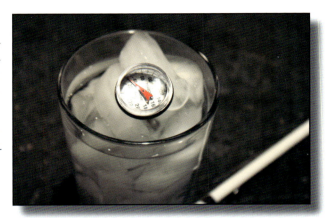

Purchase & Receiving

Always purchase your foods from a reputable vendor who is in compliance with the law. What does this mean? As a food establishment, you are required to purchase your foods from a wholesaler such as a plant that manufactures, packages, or stores foods to sell to food establishments. You as a food establishment may not get your food from another food establishment such as a restaurant, caterer, or market.

Once you have purchased your food, it's time to receive it. Again, this is where you need to begin paying attention to all the causes of foodborne illness as now the food is in your possession and it's up to you to keep it safe. You must identify all Potentially Hazardous Foods or Time/Temperature for Controlled for Safety foods (PHF/TCS) as these must be inspected carefully. You should make sure deliveries are scheduled during slow periods so your staff will have time to thoroughly inspect the food as it comes in. The most important things to remember are:

1. Cold potentially hazardous food (time/temperature control for safety food) shall be received at a temperature of 41º F (5º C) or below when received. (Eggs and raw shellfish are exempt from this requirement - see below). Hot potentially hazardous food (time/temperature control for safety food) shall be received at a temperature of 135º F (57º C) or higher.
2. Raw eggs shall be received in refrigerated equipment that maintains an ambient air temperature of 45º F (7º C) or less.
3. Live shellfish may be received and stored at 45º F (7º C) and must remain in the container in which they were received.
4. Make sure to put foods (particularly PHF/TCS foods) away immediately.
5. Check the appearance, odor, color, and condition of the packaging.
6. Prevent cross contamination: don't stack the raw chicken on your lettuce shipment; keep all items separate!

Ready-to-eat, potentially hazardous food is a special concern at receiving. Because this food will not be cooked before service, pathogenic bacterial growth should be considered a significant hazard during this step for refrigerated, ready-to-eat foods.

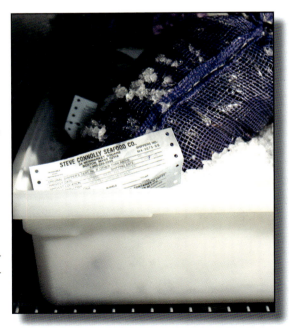

Seafood, whether ready-to-eat or not, requires special attention during receiving. For fish that are intended to be consumed raw or partially cooked, parasites are of particular concern. Because of this, they must be frozen to -31ºF (-35ºC) for at least 15 hours or -4ºF(-20ºC) for at least 7 days by either you or the seafood processor. If frozen by the processor, you should ask to see documentation that the fish has been frozen properly. Fresh fish should be firm and should not have a "fishy" odor.

As for the live shellfish, they must be live and must arrive with the shellstock identification tags attached to the containers. These tags must remain attached to the container until the container is empty. Once the container is empty, the shellstock tags must be maintained on file for 90 days.

All dry goods must be received in good condition: do not accept torn or damaged packaging or cans that are dented, swollen or rusted.

All produce must be fresh and show no evidence of spoilage such as mold, slime or odor. Also, any produce that is bruised or shows signs of pests must be rejected.

Meat and poultry should only be received if they have the United States Department of Agriculture (USDA) inspection stamps. Again, pay attention to color and texture. Frozen food must be received frozen. Any evidence of thawing (ice crystals, ice or water puddles) is reason to reject these items.

Eggs shall be clean and shells should be intact.

Liquid eggs and milk must be pasteurized.

Storage

All food and equipment must be stored properly to prevent contamination. In general, the following are guidelines to help you store everything properly:

1. Store all food and equipment at least 6 inches off the floor. This does not apply to waterproof containers such as beer kegs, bottles or cans, or milk containers in plastic crates that are stored on a clean and dry floor.
2. All food and equipment must be stored in a clean and dry area that is not exposed to splashes, dust or any other contaminants. Food and equipment may not be stored in locker rooms, toilet rooms, dressing rooms, mechanical rooms or under sewer lines, leaking pipes or any other sources of possible contamination.
3. Food should be rotated using the First In First Out system (FIFO). FIFO means the first product that you put in storage should be the first product you take out. This way you assure the oldest items are used first and the newest items are used last.
4. Food must be stored away from all chemicals, cleaning tools and supplies, and personal belongings.
5. All food must be stored either in their original sealed containers or in food grade containers that have been properly cleaned and sanitized.
6. All food in storage must be covered or tightly wrapped to prevent contamination.
7. Any food in storage that is not easily identifiable must be labeled.
8. Discard any product that has passed the manufacturers expiration date.

Cold Storage (Refrigerators and Freezers)

When food is in cold storage, one of the most important requirements is maintaining product temperature at 41º F (5º C) or lower to limit the growth of pathogenic bacteria. Refrigerator temperatures should be 38º F or 39º F (3.3º C - 3.9ºC) degrees to maintain proper product temperatures. Make sure that you monitor the temperature of the products inside these units as well as the air temperatures.

Refrigerators also need air flow to keep the entire unit cold. Do not over-crowd the refrigerator as it will interfere with air flow and cooling. Do not use solid shelves and do not line your open wire shelving with foil as this restricts airflow and cooling as well.

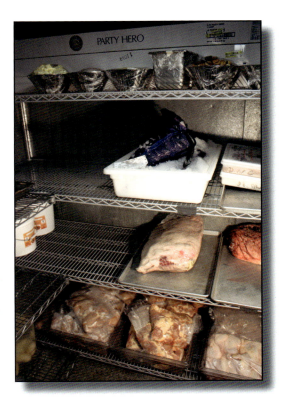

Your freezer should maintain a temperature of 0º F (-18ºC) and all food in freezers should be frozen solid.

Keep in mind that the amount of time that food is in storage is as important as maintaining proper product temperatures. PHF's/TCS ready-to-eat foods may be stored in a refrigerator that is able to maintain product temperatures at 41º F (5º C) or lower for up to 7 days. To be assured that this is being done, all PHF's/TCS ready-to-eat foods that are prepared on site should be labeled with either: the date or day by which the food shall be consumed, sold, or discarded.

Another very important requirement is storing food to prevent cross-contamination. All raw animal foods must always be stored below any ready-to-eat foods. To prevent cross contamination, the following is the proper order for how to store foods in cold storage from top to bottom: ready-to-eat foods; whole fish; whole cuts of beef or pork; ground meats and fish; and last whole or ground poultry. To further minimize the chances of cross contamination, all food should be covered and stored in food grade containers. Frozen, commercially processed and packaged raw animal foods may be stored or displayed with or above frozen commercially processed and packaged ready-to-eat foods.

Dry Storage

Dry storage should be cool, dry and well ventilated. The ideal temperature is between 50º F (10ºC) and 70º F (21º C). The ideal humidity of your dry storage area is between 50% and 60%. Store foods away from the wall and at least 6" off the floor. Utilize the FIFO stock rotation.

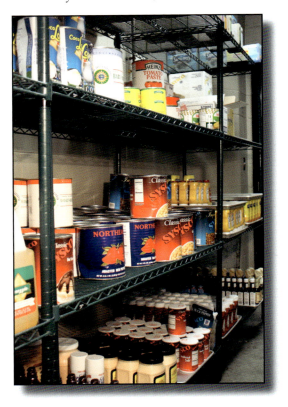

Food packaged in a food establishment must be labeled with the following: the common name of the food, or, if made from two or more ingredients, a list of ingredients in descending order; the quantity of contents; the name and place of business of the manufacturer, packer or distributor; and the name of the food source for each major food allergen (as described in Chapter 3) contained in the food. Also make sure that dating information on packaged food is not concealed. For example, price tags or other stickers may not be placed over expiration or use-by dates.

Preparation

Preparation is the step in the flow of food where you will begin working with and handling the food. This step can include thawing, washing, cutting, stuffing and breading. If food is not handled properly during preparation, food can become contaminated and possibly lead to a foodborne illness outbreak. That is why it is important to understand and address the major causes of foodborne illness: time temperature abuse; cross contamination and poor personal hygiene as they relate to preparation.

Controlling Time Temperature Abuse

As we learned in Chapter 3, it is important to keep Potentially Hazardous Foods (PHF) Time/Temperature Control for Safety Foods (TCS) out of the danger zone as much as possible. As mentioned in this chapter, the maximum time that PHF's/TCS may remain between 41º F (5º C) and 135º F (57º C) is 4 hours - this is referred to as the "Four Hour Rule". During preparation, the steps that often lead to time/temperature abuse are thawing and prepping foods that will be cooked or consumed at a later time.

Thawing

Preparation often begins with thawing frozen foods. There are only four ways to safely thaw PHF/TCS foods.

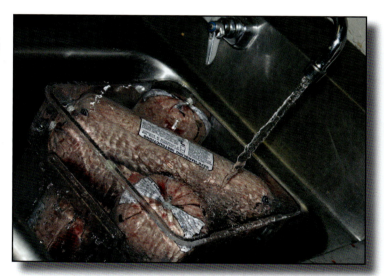

1. Thaw food in the refrigerator. As long as the refrigerator can maintain product temperatures at 41º F (5º C) degrees or lower the food will never enter the temperature danger zone.
2. Thaw food under cold running water - water temperature must be 70º F (21º C) degrees or lower, the food must be fully submerged, and the water must be continually flowing. Ready-to-eat foods that are thawing under cold running water may not exceed 41º F (5º C).
3. Thaw food in the microwave as long as it goes immediately into the cooking process. Microwaves can not be used to thaw products that will be cooked at a later time.
4. Thaw food as part of the cooking process. This is often done for products like chicken tenders that are taken from the freezer and are immediately put in the fryer or frozen ravioli that is put into boiling water directly from the freezer.

Other Time/Temperature Issues

Now unless you are working in a kitchen preparation area that is 41º F (5º C) or lower (most kitchens are not!) the temperature of foods will often enter the temperature danger zone as you are working with it. It is important to minimize the time food is in the temperature danger zone because bacteria will begin growing anytime food is between 41º F (5º C) and 135º F (57º C) degrees. Minimizing time in the danger zone can be done by:
1. Preparing food in small batches.
2. Only working on one product or performing one step at a time.
3. Putting food back into the cooler that is not being actively prepared.
4. Using ice baths for PHF/TCS foods while you are preparing the product.
5. Pre-cooling canned goods like tuna and mayonnaise before using them in products such as tuna salad or sandwiches.

The Food Code technically allows cold PHF/TCS to be in the danger zone up to 6 hours as long as the food remains under 70º F (21º C). If the food goes over 70º F (21º C) you have only 4 hours. Food must be discarded after either limit is reached. Beware that most jurisdictions will not allow this form of time temperature control without variances and detailed HACCP plans and some will not allow it at all. (See Time as a Public Health Control on page 42.)

Guidelines for Preparing Specific Food Items

Produce

All fruits and vegetables must be washed and dried before they are cut, cooked or combined with other food ingredients. Make sure that only safe potable drinking water is used to wash fruits and vegetables. Always keep washed vegetables separate from unwashed vegetables and any raw meat, poultry or seafood during storage and preparation.

Remember that cut melons, tomatoes and leafy greens are PHF/TCS foods and must be kept at 41º F (5 º C) or lower to control bacterial growth.

Establishments serving "Highly Susceptible Populations" or " High Risk Populations" such as day care centers and nursing homes cannot serve raw seed sprouts.

Eggs, Egg or Milk Batters, Breading

Store batters containing milk and eggs on ice if possible and always take them out in small batches. Determine the standard for discarding batter or breading, perhaps discarding after each batch or at the end of a shift.

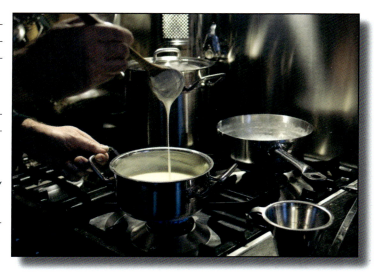

Due to the increasing number of people with food allergies and cross contamination issues, separate batters/breading should be used for each product.

Again, establishments classified by the local board of health as primarily serving "High Risk Populations" must use pasteurized eggs in meals that will not be cooked thoroughly or contain raw eggs such as Caesar salad dressing or Hollandaise sauce. Although it is not required, all establishments should consider using pasteurized eggs for these meals as well.

Pooled eggs should be cooked immediately or kept at 41°F (5 ºC) or lower during preparation and storage.

Never combine different batches of pooled eggs, batters or breading and make sure that containers are always cleaned and sanitized between different batches.

Salads Containing PHF/TCS Foods

Pasta, potato, chicken and tuna salad can be very dangerous if not handled properly- and as you read earlier it's not because of the mayo! These salads are often made from "leftover" products so it is very important that specific procedures have been followed for cooking, cooling and storing the potentially hazardous items before they are used for salads. (See Cooking, Cooling and Holding later in this chapter). Make sure that salads are discarded after seven days from when the original PHF/TCS product was cooked/cooled - not the date the salad was made. This is, of course, providing that the salad has maintained 41 degrees or lower.

Fresh Squeezed Juice

Juice that is going to be packaged on site for sale must be treated to reduce or eliminate the presence of pathogens by implementing and following an approved HACCP plan.

By law, if the juice has not been pasteurized it must be labeled with the following statement according to federal regulations.:

"WARNING: This product has not been pasteurized and, therefore, may contain harmful bacteria that can cause serious illness in children, the elderly, and persons with weakened immune systems."

Ice

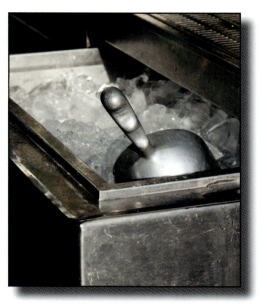

Many people don't realize that ice is food. Proper procedures must be followed to handle ice.
1. Ice must always be made from safe, potable drinking water.
2. Ice that has been used for cooling food cannot be used as an ingredient or for direct consumption with beverages.
3. Only cleaned and sanitized equipment should be used for ice storage and dispensing.
4. Do not use bare hands or glass to scoop ice-always use a food grade scoop with a handle.
5. Ice scoops must be stored on a clean sanitized surface or stored in the ice with the handle completely out of the ice as it is most likely contaminated.
6. Do not store packaged beverages (such as wine bottles, milk or juice cartons) in ice that is intended for consumption.

Specific Practices That Require a Variance

There are some practices listed below that are considered high risk and may not be performed without a variance from the health department. A variance is basically like an "approval" or waiver from the local board of health to participate in a practice that is considered "high risk" or one that deviates from the local regulations. In addition to the variance, some health departments may also require you to submit and follow an approved HACCP Plan. The following practices would require a variance and possibly a HACCP plan:
1. Smoking food as a method of food preservation rather than as a method of flavor enhancement;
2. Curing food;
3. Using food additives or adding components such as vinegar as a method of food preservation rather than flavor enhancement or to render a food so that it is not potentially hazardous or TCS (for example, the preparation of sushi requires a variance);
4. Packaging food using a reduced oxygen packaging method;
5. Custom processing animals that are for personal use for food and not for sale or service in a food establishment;
6. Operating a molluscan shellfish tank used to store and display shellfish that are offered for human consumption;
7. Preparing food by another method that is determined by the regulatory authority to require a variance; or
8. Sprouting seeds or beans.

Cooking

Cooking is one of the most important steps in the flow of food. When raw meat, seafood, poultry and eggs are cooked to the proper minimum cooking temperature, harmful pathogens can be reduced to safe levels. Minimum internal cooking temperatures have been developed by the FDA for all types of foods that you will be cooking in your establishment. Since cooking is such a critical step in the process it is very important that employees take the temperature of foods they are cooking to verify that required cooking temperatures are being met. See the chart below for specific time/temperature requirements.

Some important things to remember when cooking are:
1. Always use the proper thermometer for the product being tested.
2. Always use a properly calibrated thermometer.
3. Always take the temperature in the thickest part of the product being tested.
4. Make sure thermometer is cleaned and sanitized before and after use.
5. If the product is oddly shaped (i.e. a turkey) take the temperature in a few different spots.

Many establishments have certain menu items that are served raw or may be under-cooked. Perhaps a Caesar salad dressing containing raw eggs, or raw fish in sushi, or even a burger that a customer may request rare or medium rare. These items will not reach the required minimum cooking temperature so establishments must warn the customer about the risks of consuming raw or under cooked meat, seafood, poultry and eggs through the use of a "Consumer Advisory".

There are two parts to the consumer advisory: the disclosure and the reminder statements.

The disclosure includes a description of the animal derived food such as "oysters on the half shell (raw oysters)" or "hamburgers (may be cooked to order)" or identifying the items by marking them with an asterisk referring to a footnote that states those items are served raw, undercooked, or may contain raw ingredients.

The reminder needs to include the risks associated with consuming raw or under-cooked products. The reminder can be in one of the following three formats. Contact your local regulatory agency for posting requirements and specific wording for your jurisdiction.

1. Consuming raw or undercooked meats, poultry, seafood, shellfish, or eggs may increase your risk of foodborne illness;
2. Consuming raw or undercooked meats, poultry, seafood, shellfish, or eggs may increase your risk of foodborne illness, especially if you have certain medical conditions; or
3. Regarding the safety of these items, written information is available upon request. When using this option, you must have the information available.

Microwave Cooking

If any raw animal foods will be cooked in the microwave, additional steps must be taken to ensure the safety of these items:
1. Food must be rotated or stirred throughout or midway through the cooking process;
2. Food shall be kept covered;
3. All raw animal foods must be cooked to 165° F (74° C) degrees or higher in all parts of food; and
4. Food must be allowed to stand for two minutes after cooking.

There are special requirements for Highly Susceptible Populations. In highly susceptible populations, you may not serve or offer for sale in ready-to-eat form any raw animal foods or partially cooked animal foods. All raw animal foods must be cooked to required minimum internal cooking temperatures. In addition, hamburgers on a children's menu may not be "cooked-to-order", they must be cooked to the minimal internal temperatures.

Minimum Cooking Temperatures

Food Item	Minimum Internal Temperature	Time at the Minimum Temp.
Poultry (ground or whole), wild game, stuffed fish, meat, or pasta. Any stuffing that contains meat, fish or poultry.	165° F (74°C)	15 seconds

Minimum Cooking Temperatures Cont'd

Food Item	Minimum Internal Temperature	Time at the Minimum Temp.
Raw animal foods cooked in a microwave oven.	165º F (74ºC)	Rotated or stirred during cooking to compensate for uneven distribution of heat. Cover to retain surface moisture. Allowed to stand covered for 2 minutes after cooking to attain temperature equilibrium.
Ground Beef, Ground Pork and Ground Seafood. Raw Eggs not prepared for immediate service. Injected Meats. Comminuted Commercially Raised Game. Animals and Exotic Species of Game Animals. Comminuted Fish and Meats.	The most common choice is: 155ºF (68ºC) for 15 seconds There are three other options: 158ºF (70ºC) for 1 second; 150ºF (66ºC) for 1 minute; or 145ºF (63ºC) for 3 minutes	
Fish or meat not referred to elsewhere on this table.	145ºF (63ºC)	15 seconds
Unpasteurized shell eggs prepped for immediate service.	145ºF (63ºC)	15 seconds
Fruits and vegetables, grains, rice pasta that are cooked for hot holding. Commercially processed RTE foods for hot holding.	135ºF (57ºC)	Not Specified
Roast beef rare	130º F (54.4ºC)	112 minutes There is a relationship between how long the roast is cooked and its minimum temperature see 3-401.11 of the code.
Unpasteurized shell eggs that will be placed in hot holding.	155ºF (68ºC)	

Cooling

Cooling is one of the last steps in the flow of food. It is critical that it is done properly because the food will pass through the temperature danger zone. You remember that, right? There have been many documented cases of foodborne illness caused by improper cooling methods. Sometimes it is because employees are not provided with the proper equipment, or they do not have adequate space, or they have not been properly trained. Since foods will enter the temperature danger zone during the cooling process, it is critical that employees are trained on time and temperature parameters for cooling and the different methods that can be used to help facilitate the cooling of TCS/PHF foods.

Cooling parameters:

Cooked PHF/TCS foods must be cooled from 135º F (57º C) to 70º F. (21º C) within 2 hours or less. This is a critical step because bacteria can grow rapidly between these temperatures. If time is not controlled during cooling, some bacteria may also start to produce toxins. Once the PHF/TCS food is cooled to 70º F. (21º C) you have 4 hours to get from 70º F (21º C) to 41º F (5º C).

The total cooling time is six hours provided that the food reaches 70º F (21º C) within the first two hours.

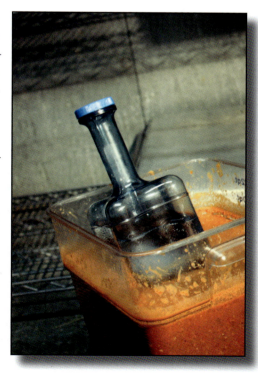

There are several things that can be done to cool foods quickly:
1. Place food in shallow pans.
2. Separate the food into smaller or thinner portions.
3. Use rapid cooling equipment such as a blast chiller.
4. Stir the food in a container placed in an ice water bath.
5. Use containers that facilitate the transfer of heat (stainless steel is a much better transfer of heat and cold than plastic).
6. Add ice as an ingredient.
7. Stir food with an ice wand.
8. Keep food uncovered or loosely covered to facilitate transfer of heat from surface of food. Make sure to protect food from overhead contamination.

Hot foods should never be placed in cold holding units such as refrigerators or freezers. These units are designed to keep cold foods cold, not to cool hot foods. There are a couple of issues when placing hot food in a refrigerator. First, studies have shown that placing hot food such as chili in a refrigerator in a large container such as a five gallon bucket can take up to four days to thoroughly cool to 41 degrees or lower. And second, placing hot food in refrigerators or freezers can also increase the ambient temperature of the unit. You can finish the cooling process in refrigerated storage once the product has cooled to 70° F. (21° C) or lower. Employees must continue to monitor products to ensure that they continue to cool to 41° F (5° C) or lower in four hours or less. Once the food has reached 41° F (5° C) or colder, make sure to cover or wrap it.

These parameters are just minimum requirements. If employees can get foods cooled faster than the time requirements listed above - even better! The less time PHF/TCS food spends in the temperature danger zone the less bacteria will grow. If these parameters are not met, food must either be discarded or re-heated to 165° F (74° C) and the cooling process must begin again.

Reheating

Reheating Foods for Hot Holding

Reheating foods that have been previously cooked is a common task in most restaurants. For most foods that are going into hot holding, you must reheat them to 165°F (74°C) for 15 seconds. Reheating must be done within 2 hours. Roasts have a slight exception to this rule as do foods that are taken from a commercially processed, hermetically sealed container. Please see the chart below.

Once the food reaches the minimum temperature for the correct time, it must be held at 135°F (57°C) or higher.

Reheating Requirements

Food Item	Minimum Temperature	Time at the Minimum Temperature	Maximum Time to Reach Temperature
Food that is cooked, cooled, and reheated	165° F (74° C)	15 seconds	2 Hours
Food that is reheated in a microwave oven	165° F (74° C)	Hold for 2 minutes	2 Hours
Food that is taken from a commercially processed, hermetically sealed container or intact package	135° F (57° C)	No time specified	2 Hours
Un-sliced portions of cooked meat roasts	Same as original cooking. There is a relationship between how long the roast is cooked and its minimum temperature see 3-401.11 of the code.	Same as original cooking. There is a relationship between how long the roast is cooked and its minimum temperature see 3-401.11 of the code.	N/A

Reheating Foods for Immediate Service

Foods that are being reheated for immediate service have no temperature requirements. Amazing, something you can do without a rule! Well, we need a rule: this can only be done if the food has been cooked and cooled according to the rules in the Cooking & Cooling sections found earlier in this chapter.

Holding

When food is held, cooled, and reheated in a food establishment, there is an increased risk from contamination caused by employees or dirty equipment. Harmful bacteria that are introduced into a product that is not held at proper temperature have the opportunity to multiply to large numbers in a short period of time. Once again, management of personal hygiene, prevention of cross-contamination, and controlling time and temperature impact the safety of the food at this point. To prevent bacterial growth when food is being held, all hot food must be held at 135º F (57º C) or above and all cold food must be held at or below 41º F (5º C). Let's talk about specific requirements:

Hot Foods:
1. Hot foods must be held so the internal temperature is at 135º F (57º C) or higher. (This is the food temperature, not the holding unit temperature).
2. Measure temperatures often, at least once every four hours. If the food drops below 135º F (57º C), it must be discarded if it has been more than four hours, or reheated if it has been less than four hours in the danger zone.
3. If the internal temperature stays above 135º F (57º C) it can be held indefinitely.

Cold Foods:
1. Cold food must be held so that the internal temperature is at 41º F (5º C) or lower. (Again, this is the food temperature, not the holding unit temperature).
2. When determining how often to check the temperature of cold food (particularly for those cold foods in display), keep in mind that it should be done often enough that corrective actions can be taken if necessary. For example, if the food is in the danger zone and your last temperature check was 6 hours ago, it must be discarded. If your food is in the danger zone and your last temperature check 2 hours ago indicated a temperature of 41º F (5º C) or less, you can put the food in an ice bath or a freezer until the temperature drops to 41º F (5º C) or less.
3. If the internal temperature of the cold food remains at 41º F (5º C) or lower, the food may be held for up to seven days.

Time as a Public Health Control

There are some situations where it is not desirable or possible to maintain these temperatures, so time (rather than temperature) must be used to protect the food from bacterial growth. As we know from information presented in chapter 3, all potentially hazardous foods (PHF's) / time temperature control for safety foods (TCH) may remain in the temperature danger zone for up to four hours. If you choose to keep foods in the danger zone for up to four hours without temperature control, you must have written procedures in place to document and verify that this is being done safely. The code requires that the food is marked or otherwise identified to indicate the time that is 4 hours past the point in time when the food is removed from temperature control.

For cold food, you actually have up to six hours. But again, there are specific requirements. The Food Code states that cold food may be held for up to 6 hours if the internal temperature always remains below 70º F (21º C). This of course assumes the food was properly held at 41º F (5º C) or cooler at all times prior to this and that the food was clearly labeled with the time it was removed from refrigerated storage.

Please be aware that your local health department may not allow for any food to ever be out of temperature control and may cite this as a critical violation.

Service & Display

Service is your last battle in preventing foodborne illness. Since you have kept it so safe through the whole receiving, storage, preparing, cooking, reheating, cooling and holding steps, lets not blow it now!

1. Everyone, including servers and bartenders, should be trained in handwashing and the illness policy outlined in Chapter 4: Personal Hygiene.
2. Serve food quickly after cooking or reheating to keep harmful pathogens (See Chapter 3 Hazards) from multiplying.
3. Never handle or serve a ready-to-eat food with bare hands. Remember that ready-to-eat foods are those that need no further cooking or washing and are now "ready to eat!" Most all foods handled by servers are ready-to-eat foods.
4. Handle all utensils, whether for serving or eating, by the handle. Avoid contact with the portion that will contact food. Only use cleaned and sanitized utensils for service. They should only be used for a single food item. (Don't dip a spoon into the green beans and then the potatoes). The utensils should be much longer than the display dishes so the contaminated handle will not touch the food. If serving utensils are stored in the food for continuous use (we call these "in-use utensils"), the handles must be out of the food. In-use utensils may also be stored on a clean and sanitized surface as long as they are cleaned and sanitized every 4 hours. You may also store in-use utensils in hot water as long as that water can be maintained at 135º F (57º C) or higher.

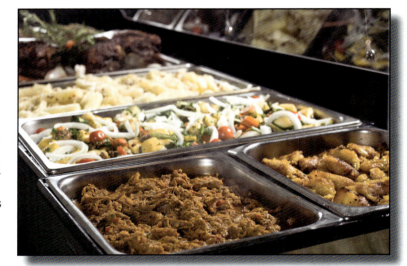

5. Do not touch the food contact surface of a plate. This is easy to do when you raise or lower a plate as the thumb naturally wants to steady the load. Don't do it.
6. Ice to be used in drinks must be handled properly because ice is food. Ice used to cool or display items can never be used for consumption.
7. Keep the amount of food that is being held for service in small batches to minimize the risk of temperature abuse.
8. You can not re-serve any food unless it is prepackaged and unopened. Examples of items you may re-serve are sugar packets, wrapped crackers, individual packets of condiments, etc. The exception to this rule is that bottled condiments like ketchup and mustard may be re-served. Keep in mind that these unopened prepackaged foods should not be reserved in highly susceptible populations. And always keep raw PHF/TCS food items separate from ready to eat foods.

Self Service

Self service items such as those in salad bars or buffets should be protected with sneeze guards no higher than 14" (36cm) above the counter that extend beyond the food by at least 7" (18cm).

The cold food must be kept at 41º F. (5º C) or below and hot foods must be kept at 135º F. (57º C) or higher. The only exception to the hot holding rule is for a whole roast of beef or pork that has been cooked to an internal temperature of 130º F (54º C). These roasts can be held at 130º F (54º C). Use thermometers regularly to check the temperatures of all your hot and cold holding items. Customers may not re-use their plates for a second (or third) trip. They must use cleaned and sanitized plates for each trip. Food can easily become contaminated when the dispensing utensil touches the customers dirty plate, then goes back into the food in the buffet or salad bar. Prepackaged foods for vending machines or self service will have labeling with the expiration date or the use by dates. Inspect these labels daily and discard any expired foods at once.

Chapter 5 - Quiz

1. Which of the following are examples of cross-contamination?
    A. An employee fails to wash her hands after cutting raw chicken and proceeds to handle hamburger buns with her bare hands.
    B. An employee stores the fruit salad under the turkey that is being thawed in the refrigerator.
    C. An employee uses a sponge to clean the cutting board that was just used to wipe down a dirty counter-top.
    D. All of the above

2. Cross contamination can be prevented by:
    A. Preparing raw food and RTE food at separate times.
    B. Cleaning and sanitizing equipment after using with raw food.
    C. Cooking food to the required minimal internal temperature.
    D. Both A and B

3. When calibrating a thermometer using the ice point method the thermometer should read _____ when submerged in the ice water.
    A. 12º F (-11º C)
    B. 31º F (-1º C)
    C. 32º F (0º C)
    D. 41º F (5º C)

4. When receiving the food, the following must ALL be received at 41 degrees or lower:
    A. Beef, poultry and whole tomatoes
    B. Beef, poultry and live shellfish
    C. Cut melon, raw shell eggs, canned tuna
    D. Fresh fish, milk, poultry

5. Shell stock tags must be kept on file for _____ from the harvest date.
    A. 7 days
    B. 21 days
    C. 41 days
    D. 90 days

6. All PHF/TCS foods must be received at 41º F (5º C) or lower with the exception of:
    A. Raw shell eggs and live shellfish.
    B. Poultry and live shellfish.
    C. Fresh whole fish and raw shell eggs.
    D. Beef and tofu.

7. The following items should be rejected during receiving:
    A. Canned goods that are severely dented
    B. Fresh seafood that has a strong "fishy" odor
    C. Poultry received at 45º F (7º C)
    D. All of the above

8. Refrigerators should not be overloaded with food because it:
    A. Makes it difficult for employees to find what they are looking for.
    B. Could damage the packages of food.
    C. Restricts air-circulation.
    D. Could break or warp the shelves in the unit.

9. Time/Temperature abuse can be controlled during preparation by all of the following except:
    A. Taking only one product out at a time.
    B. Using color-coded cutting boards.
    C. Preparing food in small batches.
    D. Storing ingredients such as egg/milk batters on ice during preparation.

10. All of the following are safe ways to thaw frozen foods except:
    A. Placing bread on the counter to thaw overnight.
    B. Placing chicken in the refrigerator to thaw.
    C. Placing burgers directly on the grill from the freezer.
    D. Thawing shrimp in a bucket of standing water.

11. The minimum cooking temperature for ground chicken is:
    A. 155º F (68º C) for 15 seconds.
    B. 140º F (60º C) for 15 seconds.
    C. 165º F (74º C) for 15 seconds.
    D. 180º F (82º C) for 15 seconds.

12. Your establishment does not serve highly susceptible populations, so meat, poultry, seafood and eggs can be served raw or undercooked provided that:
    A. The customer has been warned about the potential risks of consuming raw or undercooked foods through the use of a "consumer advisory".
    B. The PIC is the one to prepare the food.
    C. The food is treated with sanitizer to reduce bacteria to safe levels.
    D. The server evaluates the customer to determine if consuming raw food would be a good idea.

13. A small café wants to use the microwave to cook eggs for the egg sandwiches they will be serving. In order to do this safely they must:
    A. Wash the eggs before cracking.
    B. Cook the eggs to a minimum internal temperature of 165º F (74º C).
    C. Stir the eggs halfway through the cooking process and let sit for 2 minutes after cooking.
    D. Both B and C

14. When cooling a large batch of clam chowder, what has the greatest influence on getting the temperature down quickly?
    A. The quantity of the food being cooled and the type of container it is in.
    B. The ingredients and the initial temperature of the food product.
    C. The size of the pot and the temperature of the refrigerator.
    D. The size and temperature of the refrigerator.

Chapter 5 | Flow of Food | Page 46

15. The time/temperature parameters for safely cooling require cooked PHF/TCS foods to be cooled from:
    A. 135º F (57º C) to 70º F. (21º C) in 2 hours or less and then from 70º F (21º C) to 41º F (5º C) or lower in 6 more hours or less.
    B. 135º F (57º C) to 80º F. (27º C) in 2 hours or less and then from 80º F. (27º C) to 41º F (5º C) or lower in 4 more hours or less.
    C. 212º F (100º C) to 135º F (57º C) in 2 hours or less and then from 135º F (57º C) to 70º F. (21º C) or lower in 4 more hours or less.
    D. 135º F (57º C) to 70º F. (21º C) in 2 hours or less and then from 70º F. (21º C) to 41º F (5º C) or lower in 4 more hours or less.

16. A stuffed chicken breast must be hot held at a minimum temperature of:
    A. 135º F (57º C) or higher.
    B. 145º F (63º C) or higher.
    C. 155º F (68º C) or higher.
    D. 165º F (74º C). or higher.

17. Foods being reheated for immediate service must be re-heated to:
    A. Any temperature, there is no requirement
    B. 165º F (74º C). or higher.
    C. 135º F (57º C) or higher.
    D. 140º F (60º C) or higher.

18. The following practices can help keep food safe during service:
    A. Providing sneeze guards over foods on display.
    B. Providing utensils to dispense food at a buffet.
    C. Having personnel monitor self service stations.
    D. All of the above.

19. The following foods can be re-served except:
    A. Unopened package of crackers.
    B. Unopened creamer.
    C. Bottled condiments such as ketchup or mustard.
    D. Basket of rolls that will be used to make croutons.

20. You are checking the hamburgers on the grill to assure proper cooking temperatures, which of the following would be the best thermometer or probe to use:
    A. A laser thermometer
    B. A penetration probe
    C. An immersion probe
    D. An air probe

21. If you would like to use Time as a Public Health Control for cold food, the food may be held out of the temperature control as long as:
    A. The temperature remains below 70º F. (21º C).
    B. The time that the food is in the danger zone is no longer than 6 hours.
    C. The food was held at 41º F (5º C) or lower prior to leaving out of temperature control.
    D. All of the above

Answer Key
1. D   2. D   3. C   4. D   5. D   6. A   7. D   8. C   9. B   10. D
11. C   12. A   13. D   14. A   15. D   16. A   17. A   18. D   19. D   20. B   21. D

Chapter 6
Cleaning & Sanitizing

Chapter at a Glance

Cleaning Agents	47
Sanitizing Procedures	48
When to Clean	49
Warewashing Machines	49
Manual Warewashing	49
Master Cleaning Schedule	50
Quiz	51

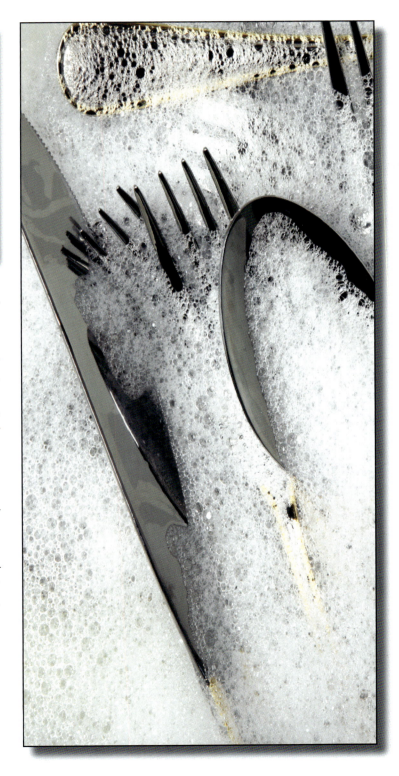

Cleaning and sanitizing have a great impact on food safety for if it is not done properly, many individuals can become ill.

Cleaning and sanitizing are two very distinct steps. Cleaning is the process that removes all food debris or soil from any item such as plates, pans, utensils, cutting boards, and just about any other surface in the kitchen. This would include floors, sinks, counters, preparation surfaces - almost anything found in a food establishment.

Cleaning Agents

There are four types of cleaning agents and each are be used for specific types of soil. There are detergents, de-greasers, acidic, and abrasive cleaning agents.

Detergents, which are used most often, are combined with hot water and are commonly used for dishes and equipment washed in a three bay sink. Detergents will loosen and lift dirt, food or grime from the surface and allow it to be rinsed away.

De-greasers are used for areas with heavy grease buildup such as floors under fryers or a ventilation hood above a grill.

Acidic cleaning agents are used for equipment where there may be a buildup of mineral deposits such as lime or calcium.

Finally, abrasive cleaning agents are most effective on surfaces where there is heavy, baked-on, cooked-on debris such as on the bottom of saute´ pans.

Sanitizing Procedures

Sanitizing is the process of killing most pathogenic micro-organisms. All food contact surfaces must be both cleaned AND sanitized. Even though something has been thoroughly cleaned, there can still be many microorganisms on the surface that can cause foodborne illness. It is important to remember that surfaces that look clean may still have germs on them that you can't see.

Sanitizing a clean surface will reduce the amount of disease-causing microorganisms (germs) to a level that is safe for humans. Sanitization can be done by one of two methods: heat or chemical. Keep in mind that sanitizing will only be effective on items that have been properly cleaned and rinsed.

To sanitize using the heat method, most high temperature warewashing machines require that the water temperature is at least 180ºF (82ºC)and is no higher than 194ºF (90ºC). You can also sanitize by heat in the three bay sink. To do this, the items must be immersed in 171ºF (77ºC) degrees water for at least 30 seconds. This is rarely done as it is difficult to maintain these water temperatures and is very difficult for employees to handle the dishes because of the very hot water.

For chemical sanitization, it is critical that the manufacturers' instructions are followed carefully. The concentration of the solution is extremely important: too much sanitizer becomes toxic to humans, too little is ineffective at killing microorganisms. The concentrations are always listed in parts per million (PPM). You must dilute the agent with water at the correct temperature (each manufacturer has specific guidelines on this depending on water hardness and pH levels). You will also need the appropriate test strips to determine the accurate PPM and a thermometer to read the temperature of the solution.

The most popular chemical sanitizers are Quats (Quaternary Ammonium Compounds), Iodine and Chlorine. Local and state regulations may require you to use or forbid the use of a particular sanitizer. (See guideline charts below for proper chemical concentrations for chemical sanitizers.)

Chlorine Solutions Guidelines

Minimum Concentration PPM	Minimum Temperatures		Exposure Time
	PH between 8-10	PH Less Than 8	
25-49	120ºF (49ºC)	120ºF (49ºC)	10 seconds
50-99	100ºF (38ºC)	75ºF (24ºC),	7 seconds
100	55ºF (13ºC)	55ºF (13ºC)	30 seconds

Quats & Iodine Solutions Guidelines

Sanitizer	Temperature	Water PH	Concentration
Iodine	75ºF (24ºC)	5 or less	12.5- 25 PPM
Quats	75ºF (24ºC)	See manufacturer specifications	See manufacturer specifications

When to Clean

You must wash, rinse, and sanitize any food contact surface including dishes, utensils, cutting boards, preparation tables, sinks, food processing equipment, food containers, glasses, prep tables, carts - anything that may come in contact with food:
1. Before each use;
2. Between uses when preparing different types of raw animal foods, such as eggs, fish, meat, and poultry;
3. Between uses when preparing ready-to-eat foods and raw animal foods, such as eggs, fish, meat, and poultry; and
4. Any time contamination occurs or is suspected.

In addition, you should periodically clean and sanitize nonfood-contact surfaces that are touched: handles, drawers, faucets, switches, controls, even trash container lids. This is another step that will keep harmful organisms from spreading to food.

Warewashing Machines

All warewashing machines must have an easily accessible and readable data plate affixed to the machine by the manufacturer that indicates the machine's design and operation specifications including:
1. Temperatures required for washing, rinsing, and sanitizing;
2. Pressure required for the fresh water sanitizing rinse; and
3. Conveyor speed for conveyor machines or cycle time for stationary rack machines.

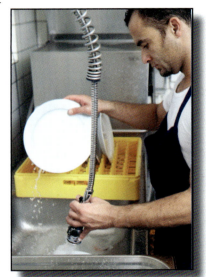

All warewashing machines must have temperature measuring devices that indicate the temperatures in both the wash and rinse tank as well as the hot water sanitizing final rinse manifold or the chemical sanitizing solution tank. Naturally, these specifications and temperature gauges do not do any good unless you follow the directions! You are required to operate warewashing machines to the manufacturers specifications. If a temperature is too low you must fix it, a speed too high, you must fix it. You get the point. If it's not working properly, you may not use the machine.

When using a warewashing machine, items need to be scraped and rinsed before being placed in the machines. Make sure that dishes and equipment are then placed on the racks so that all surfaces of the item will be exposed to the dishwashers' spray of water and sanitizer. A visual inspection of all items after sanitizing should be made and any soiled items should be run through the machine until clean. You must allow the items to air dry. Towel drying will contaminate the freshly sanitized items. Your warewashing machine needs to be cleaned just like the rest of your equipment to keep food debris from clogging spray nozzles or drains.

Manual Warewashing

Manual warewashing is a five step process. However, before you begin the five steps, the three tanks and drain boards on either side of the sink must be cleaned and sanitized.
1. Rinsing, soaking or scraping must first be done to remove most food debris from the item so that it will be easier to wash. This will also keep the wash water clear so it does not have to be changed as often.
2. The second step is washing the dishes in hot soapy water in the first tank. This will remove all

the food debris and soil. The soapy water should be at least 110°F (43° C). You should use a brush, cloth or nylon scrub pad to clean. Wash water solution should be changed when suds become low, when the water becomes dirty, or when the water becomes cold.

3. The third step is to rinse the cleaned equipment in the second tank. Rinsing in clean water will remove all detergent. This can be done by using a sprayer or dipping in the filled sink. Be sure to change rinse water when it becomes dirty or contains suds.
4. The fourth step is sanitizing. This is done in the third tank. Sanitizing in the three bay sink is usually done by using the chemical method. Make sure to follow the manufacturers instructions for the proper concentration and temperature of your sanitizing solutions.
5. Finally, the fifth step is to air dry all equipment. Place all the items upside down to drain and to air dry. Do not dry them with a towel.

After the items are dry, be sure to store them properly. All utensils should be stored with the handles up. Glasses should be stored inverted (stored with the bottoms up) so your staff can grab them without contaminating the food contact areas that will eventually touch the customers mouth. All other bowls or containers must be inverted as well.

All clean-in-place (CIP) equipment must be cleaned and sanitized as well. For electrical equipment, make sure to unplug the machine first. Disassemble the machine and remove the detachable part. These parts should be washed and sanitized in the three bay sink, ware washing machine, or according to the manufacturers instructions. You need to make sure that the cleaning and sanitizing solutions circulate throughout the piece of equipment and are able to completely drain.

Master Cleaning Schedule

Developing a master cleaning schedule for your facility is very important. This will ensure that everything will be cleaned as often as necessary. Once created, you will need to train your employees to use the schedule and monitor appropriate adherence to it. A master cleaning schedule will often have what needs to be done on a daily, weekly, monthly or even quarterly basis. It describes what needs to be cleaned, how it is to be done, and types of chemicals used. It will also often identify the person responsible for that job.

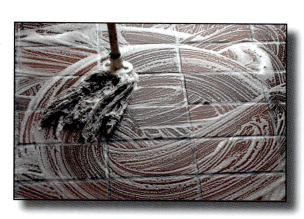

Master Cleaning Schedule format

ITEM	WHEN	HOW	SOLUTION TYPE(S)	SIGNATURE
Inside of Refrigerators	1 x week	Hot Soapy Water, Wiping Cloth	Detergent	
Kitchen Floor	Daily	Sweep with broom, mop	Floor Cleaner	
Kitchen Shelving	1 x week	Hot Soapy Water, Wiping Cloth	Detergent	
Can Opener Blade, Slicer, Mixer	Every 4 hours	Wash, rinse and sanitize	Cleanser, fresh water and sanitizer 200ppm	
Prep Tables	Every 4 hours	Wash, rinse and sanitize	Cleanser, fresh water and sanitizer 200ppm	
Ventilation Hoods	Quarterly	Professional Company	Professional Company	
Cappuccino Machine	Throughout shift, end of day	Wipe and buff exterior. Clean steamer and spout.	Hot water & Sanitizer 200 ppm.	
Ventilation Filters	1 x week	Degreaser, scrape, place in dish machine	Heavy Duty Degreaser	
Soda Nozzles	Daily	Wash, rinse and sanitize	Detergent & Sanitizer 200 ppm.	

Chapter 6 - Quiz

1. How often must "in-use" utensils be cleaned and sanitized?
    A. After each use
    B. At the end of each shift
    C. Every 4 hours when in continuous use
    D. Daily

2. Which of the following is a correct statement?
    A. All surfaces in a kitchen must be cleaned – this includes plates, pans, floors, refrigerator, forks, preparation tables and sinks.
    B. Only food contact surfaces must be cleaned.
    C. Floors, walls and ceiling must be cleaned and sanitized at the end of each day.
    D. Food contact surfaces are required to be rinsed and sanitized every four hours.

3. Your supervisor has asked that you clean the greasy ventilation hood. Which of the following would be the best cleaning agent:
    A. Chlorine
    B. A de-greaser
    C. An Abrasive cleaning agent
    D. An Acidic cleaning agent

CHAPTER 6 | CLEANING & SANITIZING | PAGE 52

4. Generally speaking, the water temperature for the sanitizing solutions must be:
   A. 41º F (5º C) -135º F (57º C)
   B. 50º F (10º C) – 70º F (21º C)
   C. 98.6º F (37º C)
   D. at the temperature specified by the manufacturer.

5. All of the following are examples of sanitizing agents except:
   A. Chlorine
   B. Acidic
   C. Iodine
   D. Quats

6. What is the third step when dishes are being washed in a three bay sink?
   A. Pre soak or scrape the dishes
   B. Sanitize the dishes
   C. Air dry the dishes
   D. Rinse the dishes in clean water

7. Which of the following should be included in a master cleaning schedule?
   A. The items to be cleaned, when they should be cleaned, how they are to be cleaned and the types of chemicals or solutions to be used.
   B. The item to be cleaned, the person responsible for cleaning the item, how the item is to be cleaned, and the reason the item needs to be cleaned.
   C. The signature of the person cleaning the item, when the items should be cleaned, what company is responsible for cleaning the item, and the temperature of the water to be used when cleaning the item.
   D. The items to be cleaned, when they should be cleaned, how they are to be cleaned, and why they are to be cleaned.

ANSWER KEY
1. C 2. A 3. B 4. D 5. B 6. D 7. A

Chapter 7
Pests

Chapter at a Glance
Identifying the Signs of Common Pests	53
Integrated Pest Management (IPM)	54
Deny Pest Entrance to Your Building	54
Prevent Access To Food, Water and Shelter	55
Hire a Professional Pest Control Operator (PCO)	55
Quiz	55

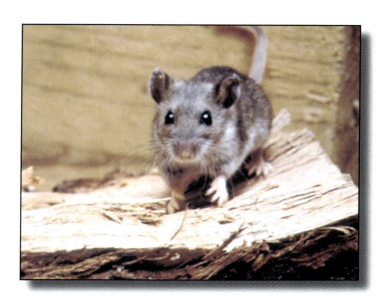

Pests are bad for business, period. Imagine a customer seeing one, imagine your restaurant on the local newscast showing some rats parading in your dining room behind closed doors. Pests can have a devastating effect on your business. Keeping them out and getting rid of the ones inside is what this chapter is all about. Insects and rodents are your main enemies and include mice, rats, flies, ants, and cockroaches. Birds, bats and countless other nasty little critters can be lumped in as well.

Pests walk over food, leave droppings and urinate on food contact surfaces, and spread disease and illness wherever they are found.

Identifying the Signs of Common Pests

First, lets try to identify the pests we are trying to prevent. Cockroaches are about 1/2"- 2" long, medium to dark brown and fairly flat. They will scatter when disturbed by light. They have a strong oily odor, their feces look like course grains of pepper, their egg casings are about the size of a grain of rice and look like a puffed rice cereal ...mmmm tasty.

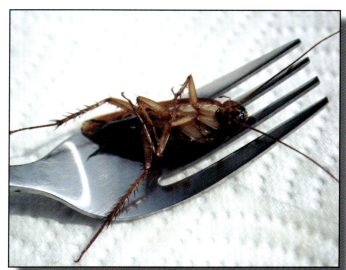

Mice and rats - everyone knows one when they see one. However, you don't have to see one to know you have a problem. Look for droppings (mice droppings are dark and about the size of rice, rats naturally have slightly larger droppings). Rodents will also leave a trail by dragging their tail through their own urine. This shows up a fluorescent green under a black light or is visible to the naked eye on a dusty surface. Shredded paper is another sign of rodents as they will gnaw at food packaging, cardboard or wood to get access to food or to create shelter.

Integrated Pest Management (IPM)

Integrated Pest Management (IPM) is the key to dealing with pests. IPM is a combined effort between you and your pest control company. It will include many of the sanitary tasks you perform on a daily basis as well as prevention and control measures implemented by your pest control company. We also call a pest control company a "Pest Control Operator" (PCO). An Integrated Pest Management plan is very simple with 3 main components:

1. Preventing pests from entering the building;
2. Preventing pests from accessing food, water and shelter for nesting or hiding; and
3. Hiring a licensed Pest Control Operator (PCO) who will also eliminate any pests that are found in your facility.

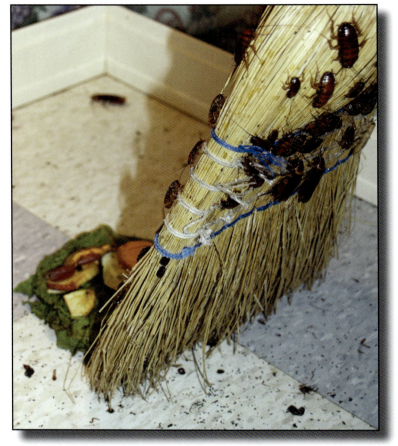

Deny Pests Entrance to Your Building

Pests can get into your establishment through cracks, gaps, or openings no matter how small. A full grown mouse needs less than 1/4" to squeeze through an opening, insects need much less space.

To prevent pests from entering:
1. Fill all cracks and holes, check for gaps around pipes that enter the building and seal around all vents, pipes, windows and door openings with sealants recommended by your PCO;
2. Screen off all vent openings;
3. Keep doors closed, install self closing devices;
4. Screen all windows that will be open with a 16 mesh to 25.4 mm (16 mesh to 1 inch); and
5. Install appropriate air curtains to control flying insects.

Pests can be brought in when food and supplies are delivered. Inspect all shipments carefully and make sure to reject all deliveries when there are signs of pests. Also, make sure to use reputable vendors who also have an IPM program.

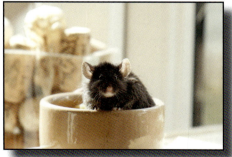
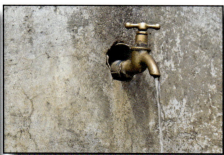
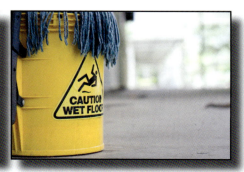

Prevent Pest Access to Food, Water and Shelter

Pests that have a continuous supply of food, water and shelter will never leave, so you must deny them these basic necessities. One of the most effective ways to deny them these necessities is to clean. (See Chapter 6: Cleaning and Sanitizing). The little hard to reach places under your equipment are not hard to reach for a mouse or a cockroach. The food debris and grease remaining in these areas are a significant food source for all types of pests. Dirty trash cans, equipment, sinks, drains, etc. . . are also of concern and must be cleaned regularly.

You must also make sure that all your food is stored properly. It must be 6 inches off the floor and, ideally, 6 inches away from the wall. All food in storage must be in covered containers or must be tightly wrapped. In addition, trash and garbage are a sources of food and shelter for pests. Keep trash/garbage receptacles covered when not in continuous use. Remove trash/garbage as often as necessary to prevent accumulation of excessive and keep those trash/garbage receptacles clean.

As for the water, do not allow water to pool in any areas. If spray methods for cleaning are used, make sure water is squeegeed down the drain. If there are any broken pipes or leaking plumbing, repair and/or replace them. Condensation from refrigerator units or air conditioning units are also a source of water.

Finally, any items that are not needed for the operation of your establishment should be removed from the premises. For example, old receipts, holiday decorations, clothing and equipment are excellent hiding places for pests. Get rid of them!

Hire a Professional Pest Control Operator (PCO)

A licensed PCO is a key component of your IPM plan. Look for a company that will inspect your building and come up with an integrated plan to control pests in your facility. A good company will work with you and use a combination of methods to help prevent and control your pests. Sometimes, this may include fixing some of those cracks and holes that are allowing pests to enter your business or giving you advice on to how to identify and eliminate conditions favorable to pests. Using pesticides should always be the last resort. If pesticides are used, they should only be used by a licensed, trained PCO.

If any insect control devices are used, they should be designed so that they retain the insect within the device. They should not be located over food preparation areas and any dead insects or insect fragments should not be able to fall into food, clean equipment, utensils, linens, and unwrapped single-service and single-use articles.

A good company will also leave a log book for you and your employees to use to document pest sightings so that they can do their job more effectively. After you've had a visit from your PCO, ask them to review their findings and suggestions with you. Pest control companies that come and go without ever communicating with you are not working in your best interests.

Chapter 7 - Quiz

1. All of the following are signs of rodent activity except:
    A. Shredded paper and cloth.
    B. Strong oily odor.
    C. Gnawing marks on food packaging.
    D. Dark rice like droppings.

2. Pests are a problem in food service establishments because:
   A. They can contaminate food and spread disease.
   B. They are distracting to employees.
   C. They eat too much food thus affecting food costs.
   D. They create a tripping hazard.

3. You can deny pests access to the establishment by:
   A. Keeping the doors of the establishment locked.
   B. Sealing any cracks, holes or other openings around the building.
   C. Keeping all food stored above the floor and in covered containers.
   D. Repairing all pipes that are leaking.

4. You can deny pests food and water by all of the following except:
   A. Covering all trash cans containing food residue when not in use.
   B. Cleaning under and behind all equipment.
   C. Emptying out all sinks, sanitize buckets and mop buckets at the end of the night.
   D. Checking deliveries for evidence of pests.

5. The following are signs of a cockroach infestation:
   A. Droppings that look like brown rice, gnawed packages of food and small nests made of old coffee filters.
   B. A strong oily smell, droppings that look like course grains of pepper and egg casings that look like puffed rice.
   C. All of the above
   D. None of the above

6. Integrated Pest Management is a combined effort between your Pest Control Operator and:
   A. Your cleaning company
   B. You and your employees
   C. The Health Department
   D. The FDA, the USDA and the CDC

7. The most important element for an effective IPM program is:
   A. Deny them food, water and shelter.
   B. Deny them from accessing your establishment.
   C. Hire a pest control operator.
   D. All of the above

ANSWER KEY
1. B   2. A   3. B   4. D   5. B   6. B   7. D

Chapter 8
Facilities & Equipment

Chapter at a Glance

Floors, Walls and Ceilings	57
Equipment & Utensils	58
Handwashing Stations	58
Water, Sewer and Plumbing	59
Refuse	60
Ventilation	60
Lighting	60
Facility Design / Plan Review	61
Maintenance	62
Quiz	62

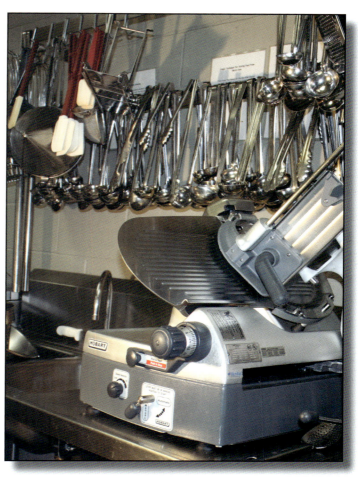

Many of the food safety practices we've discussed in the previous chapters would be nearly impossible to execute without your facilities and equipment being in compliance with the Food Code as well. So, we'll start with the basics - floors, walls and ceilings.

Floors, Walls and Ceilings:

According to the Food Code, "floors, floor coverings, walls, wall coverings, and ceilings shall be designed, constructed, and installed so they are smooth and easily cleanable". Materials must also be durable to withstand continuous traffic and repeated scrubbing.

Floors and walls of all food storage, prep and cooking areas should be non-absorbent and include a tightly sealed "coving" where the wall meets the floor. This curved transition from wall to floor, is much easier to keep clean than the typical 90 degree junction of the floor and wall.

As carpeting is not easily cleanable, it is not allowed in any food preparation area, storage area, restroom, dish washing area or kitchen - pretty much anywhere in your establishment except the dining room.

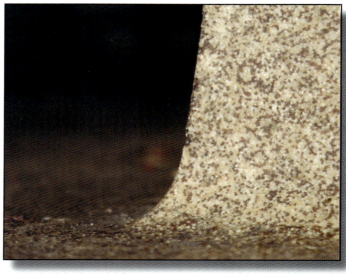

Equipment & Utensils

"Equipment and utensils" basically means anything not permanently attached to the floors, walls and ceilings. This would include "food contact surfaces," and "non-food contact surfaces."

Food contact surfaces are types of equipment with surfaces that may touch food in your establishment. These surfaces not only include cutting boards, plates, glasses, and utensils, but any other equipment you use for preparing and cooking the food. All food contact surfaces should be: smooth, easy to clean, and durable; should not have any open seams, sharp edges, cracks, chips, inclusions, pits, or similar imperfections; should be free of sharp internal angles, corners, and crevices; and should be finished to have smooth welds and joints.

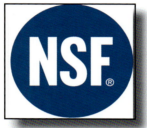 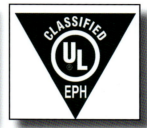 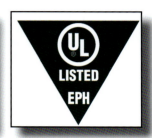

Nonfood-contact surfaces are any surface that do not touch food directly. These could include a refrigerator; storage shelves, an oven, or shelves under preparation tables.

According to the FDA, all "equipment and utensils shall be designed and constructed to be durable and to retain their characteristic qualities under normal use conditions." For example, cutting boards, food containers or even knives must be able to be used, cleaned and sanitized without falling apart or breaking.

In addition, all equipment must be stored in a manner to prevent contamination and may not be stored in any locations such as in restrooms, locker rooms, under sewer lines, leaking pipes, or near any other source of contamination. All floor mounted equipment must be at least 6 inches off the floor or sealed to the floor. Any table-based equipment must be 4 inches off the table. These requirements are primarily for ease in cleaning under the equipment.

You can be assured that your equipment meets all the FDA standards if the equipment has been approved by the National Sanitation Foundation (NSF) or Underwriters Laboratories, Inc. (UL). The NSF and UL (or more specifically UL EPH which is Underwriters Laboratories, Inc for Environmental and Public Health) approval mark on equipment means that the equipment has met or exceeded their standards as food equipment. You must use equipment that is specifically designed for commercial food service use and have the NSF and/or UL EPH approvals.

Handwashing Stations

As for personal hygiene, there is nothing more important than your handwashing stations for food safety. They should be in convenient and multiple locations near food prep, dispensing and warewashing areas and must be in or adjacent to the restrooms. They should always be clean and well stocked with supplies. Handwashing stations must have:

1. Hot and cold running water - the hot water should be at least 100º F. (38º C);
2. Soap (can be any type - bar, powdered, liquid or foaming);
3. Hand drying capabilities - disposable, single use paper towels or a warm air dryer;
4. A waste container for the paper towels; and
5. Signage - a sign that states, "Employees must wash their hands beforereturning to work". This sign must be in all languages spoken by your employees.

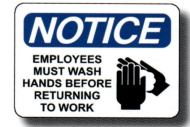

Keep in mind that hand washing sinks may only be used for hand washing (do not ever wash or rinse food or any type of equipment in these sinks) and may not be blocked or obstructed in any way at any time.

WAREWASHING MACHINES

As indicated in Chapter 6, Cleaning and Sanatizing, all warewashing machines must have an easily accessible and readable data plate affixed to the machine by the manufacturer that indicates the machine's design and operation specifications. In addition, all warewashing machines must have NSF and UL certification. It is important that these machines, just like any other equipment, are on legs at least 6 inches off the floor.

WATER, SEWER AND PLUMBING

Every food establishment needs to supply potable (drinkable) water. The approved sources of water are:

1. A public water system (your town or city's water supply);
2. A private water system that is constructed, maintained, tested and operated according to law;
3. Bottled water purchased from an approved source;
4. Closed water containers that are portable; and
5. Commercial water transport vehicles.

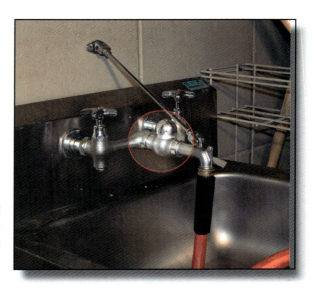

If you use a well as your water supply, you must test it according to your local jurisdictions requirements. Most regions require once a year testing and the records for those tests should be kept on file.

CROSS CONNECTIONS

Although plumbing may not appear to be a "food safety issue", it must be addressed as there are a few plumbing issues that can cause big problems. The biggest issue is the contamination of the potable water with the waste water, a problem called a "cross connection".

A common way a cross connection can occur is by having a nozzle (such as those at the end of a spray hose in the warewashing area) hang down into the sink below the flood rim. If the sink is filled with water, the water can be siphoned into the faucet contaminating the potable water supply. The best way to prevent this is to have an "air gap" which is the distance from the flood rim of the sink to the low point of the faucet outlet.

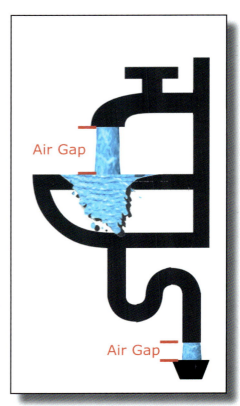

This air gap must be at least twice the diameter of the water supply inlet but never less than 1 inch (25 mm). There should also be an indirect connection such as an air gap or air break between the sink drain and floor drain for sinks used for food preparation and warewashing.

Another common way a cross connection is created is by attaching one end of a hose to a faucet with the other end submerged in a bucket. Just like siphoning gas out of a gas tank, the contaminated water from the bucket can get sucked back into your main water system. The best way to prevent this is to install a backflow device at the faucet.

Backflow prevention devices must be installed when an air gap cannot be used, as when hoses are attached to faucets. This is often seen at mop sinks. A backflow device will prevent the contaminated water from flowing into the water supply. All backflow devices must be professionally installed.

At least one service sink (also called a mop or utility sink) or curbed facility with floor drain must be provided and conveniently located for the cleaning of mops or similar wet floor cleaning tools and for the disposal of mop water and similar liquid waste.

You must provide at least one toilet, or the minimum allowed by your jurisdiction. And, it must remain in good working order. All doors to restrooms must be tight-fitting and self-closing if open to food preparation or storage. Remember, any back-up of sewage is cause for immediate closure and notifying the health department.

Overhead pipes for waste, sprinkler, gas or water in food storage, prep, dispensing areas may leak or create condensation that can drip on the food and should be avoided or shielded against this.

Refuse

Refuse is the prime attraction for rodents and other pests in your facility. Proper storage of refuse will reduce the likelihood of a pest infestation. Refuse is defined by the FDA as solid waste not carried by water through the sewage system. This includes: materials that contain food residue, recyclables, and returnables.

Indoor receptacles must be durable, cleanable, insect and rodent-resistant, leakproof, and nonabsorbent. If they contain food debris, they must be covered at all times unless they are in continuous use. If these are placed outside, they must have tight fitting lids. Remember, these must be cleaned often as dirty garbage cans attract pests. It's a good idea to use plastic liners, but these liners may not be used without a closed receptacle.

Outdoor refuse, recyclables, and returnables must have tight fitting lids, doors or covers. In some situations, they may need to be locked. They should be located on a dry, non-absorbing surface sloped to a drain and stored so that they are inaccessible to insects and rodents. If these containers have drains, the plugs must be in place.

In terms of outer building openings, such as doors and windows, they must be protected against the entry of vermin by filling or closing holes and gaps along floors, walls, and ceiling; by having tight fitting windows and solid, self-closing, tight fitting doors; and by equipping door or window openings with 16 mesh screens or air curtains. The "mesh" in the screen refers to the number of holes per square inch.

Ventilation

The purpose of ventilation systems is to remove heat, steam, condensation, vapors, smoke and fumes from food preparation and warewashing areas. Exhaust ventilation hood systems in food preparation and warewashing areas include components such as hoods, fans, guards, and duct work. These shall be designed to prevent grease or condensation from draining or dripping onto food or any type of equipment. The filters must be easily removed for replacement and cleaning, which must be done regularly. Check with your local jurisdiction and fire codes regarding service and cleaning requirements.

Lighting

All areas in a food establishment must have sufficient lighting for safety and sanitation purposes. For obvious reasons, areas where food is being prepared must have more lighting than areas such as dining rooms and restrooms. In addition to lighting requirements as outlined below, all lights should have shatter resistant bulbs or protective covers that will prevent glass from dropping in or on food accidently. The following is a schedule of required lighting intensity as measured in "foot candles". A foot candle is a measurement of lighting intensity.

Lighting Levels Required by the Food Code

Minimum Lighting Levels	Area of Application
108 lux (10 foot candles) at a distance of 75 cm (30 inches) above the floor	Dry storage
	Refrigerated or frozen walk-in storage
	All other areas while cleaning such as dining areas
215 lux (20 foot candles)	Reach-in refrigerators and freezers
	Buffet service, salad bars or any other self service areas
	Restrooms, handwashing stations, and warewashing areas
	Utensil storage areas
540 lux (50 foot candles)	Food preparation areas, particularly in areas where there is dangerous equipment such as slicers, grinders, band saws, and knives

Facility Design / Plan Review

Although the actual structure of a food service establishment is not something that is thought about on a daily basis, the physical facilities and layout of the establishment play a very important role in keeping your food safe.

When beginning the kitchen design, it is important to keep in mind the layout and location of all storage areas, food prep areas, warewashing areas, cooking areas, and serving areas. For example, all cold storage areas should be near food preparation areas to help maintain time temperature requirements. Garbage and recycling areas must be separate from food storage areas to prevent cross-contamination. Multiple hand washing stations are a must to help employees comply with personal hygiene regulations for washing hands. A well designed kitchen makes it much easier to comply with all of the regulations that we have been talking about in this book.

Most health departments require a "plan review" to make sure that the kitchen is not only well designed, but is also in compliance with the food code. In addition, the health department will want to ensure that all equipment meets FDA requirements, that the proposed menu can be prepared safely in the kitchen, that all plumbing and electrical wiring meets building codes, and that the construction materials selected for the floors walls and ceilings are durable and easily cleaned. Some health departments may also want to know about employee training, illness policies, and companies to be used for pest control, servicing of hoods and grease traps, and general maintenance of equipment.

These "Plan Reviews" are required to be submitted to the local health department for review and approval before:
1. The construction of a food establishment;
2. The conversion of an existing structure for use as a food establishment; or
3. The remodeling of a food establishment or a change of type of food establishment.

Again, you must contact your local health department BEFORE any construction begins! Starting construction before plans have been approved can be disastrous. We have had many clients who have completed the construction and then submitted plans to the health department only to find out that their establishment does not meet code. In these situations, they have had to demolish the new construction and begin again.

Maintenance

This is simple - keep the facility and all equipment well maintained. Part of maintenance means cleaning regularly which was addressed in chapter 6 "Cleaning & Sanitizing." Keeping the facility clean (inside and out) will also help control pests. All mechanical equipment from refrigerators to mixers to hoods must be serviced regularly in order for them to work properly and safely. The building itself must be inspected for leaks, cracks, and holes that may allow pests to find a new home.

Chapter 8 - Quiz

1. According to the FDA, floors must be:
    - A. Smooth and easily cleanable.
    - B. Made with materials that are durable.
    - C. Covered with carpeting.
    - D. Both A and B above.

2. Coving is required in any areas where food is being prepared. Coving:
    - A. Is the curved transition from the wall to the floor.
    - B. Is the type of material used for floors, walls and ceilings.
    - C. Is the material that is used between the tiles to keep them in place.
    - D. Refers to the coverings on ceiling tiles.

3. Food may be stored in which of the following areas:
    - A. In a locker room with supplies of toilet paper.
    - B. In a dry storage room with equipment.
    - C. Under sewer lines.
    - D. Under the shelves where chemicals are stored.

4. You can be assured that your equipment meets FDA standards if you see the following stamped or embossed on equipment:
    - A. CDC
    - B. USDA
    - C. NSF
    - D. ROP

5. Handwashing stations do not require:
    - A. Hot and cold running water.
    - B. Soap.
    - C. A clock.
    - D. A waste container.

6. All water used for drinking, washing dishes and food preparation must be potable. What does this mean?
   A. That the water comes from a well
   B. That the water is safe and drinkable
   C. That the water can be used to scrub pots
   D. All of the above

7. An employee needs to dump the mop water, which sink should he use?
   A. The three bay sink
   B. The hand washing sink
   C. The food preparation sink
   D. The utility sink

8. All areas in a food service establishment must have enough lighting so that employees can do their work safely. How much lighting is required in an area where there are slicers and knives?
   A. 50 Watts
   B. 20 lux
   C. 10 foot candles
   D. 50 foot candles

9. A plan review is required before construction of a kitchen begins. This plan review should include:
   A. Specification sheets for all equipment so the health department is assured that the equipment meets FDA requirements.
   B. A copy of the proposed menu.
   C. Confirmation from the building department that all electrical and plumbing meets building codes.
   D. All of the above

Answer Key
1. D   2. A   3. B   4. C   5. C   6. B   7. D   8. D   9. D

Chapter 9
Active Managerial Control

Chapter at a Glance

Training   65

HACCP   66

Quiz   70

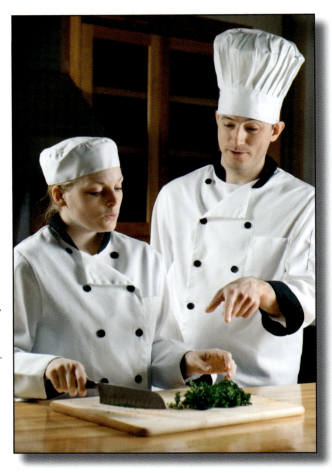

The FDA uses the term "Active Managerial Control" to describe the industry's responsibility for developing and implementing food safety management systems to prevent, eliminate, or reduce the occurrence of foodborne illness risk factors. Basically, this means that the person in charge (PIC) must take an active role in preventing foodborne illness. Based on the risk factors for foodborne illness, the PIC must be able to:

1. Demonstrate knowledge in food safety;
2. Have all employees adhere to strict hygienic practices and have an illness policy;
3. Control time and temperature for potentially hazardous foods;
4. Prohibit bare hand contact with ready to eat foods and;
5. Have a consumer advisory for any raw or undercooked animal foods offered for sale or service.

Specific elements of an effective food safety management system may include developing "Standard Operating Procedures" (SOPs). These are written operational steps that can be developed for various types of processes conducted in a food establishment. For example, they may be written for a food preparation process such as proper thawing of foods. These may be written for proper cleaning and sanitizing, for purchasing specifications, for monitoring and record keeping, or even for hand washing.

A key element in food safety management systems is training all managers and employees. This is essential to assure that all the standards are being met. An establishment cannot operate safely if the employees are not aware of or do not understand their responsibilities.

An effective food safety management system may include developing a HACCP (Hazard Analysis Critical Control Point) plan which is also a written document (which will be discussed in more detail below) to assist management with food safety.

Training

Now that you have learned everything you need to know about how to serve food safely, you must train your staff. This is not always easy as there are many training methods and people learn in different ways. Add language and cultural barriers and you are in for an even more daunting task. I would begin with all your existing employees. What do they know? What do they need to know to do their job safely? The difference between these two is the "training gap" that you need to fill. Remember, not all employees are required to know all aspects of food safety at your establishment - that's your job. They are required to be trained in food safety as it relates to their assigned duties. If there are language barriers, see if you can get a translator to help with the training. Often, family members who are bilingual are more than happy to help if it helps their mother, father, or brother keep their job and do their job better.

You may want to begin training by using "classroom style" training. This means sitting down with your employees with this book and reviewing all the important concepts such as proper personal hygiene, time and temperature control, how to prevent cross-contamination, and how to clean and sanitize properly. You should review how each of these issues can be conducted in your business. Don't assume your employees already know this - you'll be surprised by what they don't know. I strongly recommend that this training be conducted while you are not open for business so you and your staff will be able to focus on the material being covered. I also recommend going around your establishment after this training and having your employees 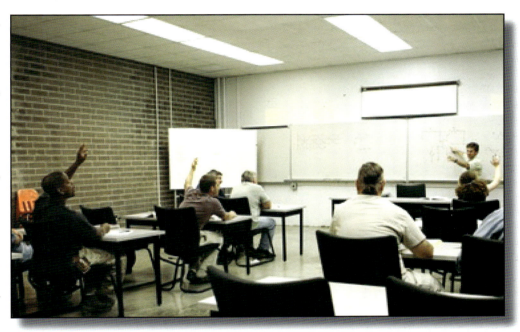 point out what is being done correctly and areas in need of improvement. This can actually be turned into a game. Break up your staff into two groups - the group that can come up with the most suggestions on how to improve your food safety would win. What they win is up to you.

Many food safety trainers offer this type of training and many call it Food Safety 101 or a food handlers class. Many restaurants say that their employees sometimes need to hear this from someone outside the restaurant in order for them to listen and to take the information being presented seriously.

In addition, and perhaps more importantly, any new employees hired from here on out should be trained in food safety before they are allowed to handle or serve any food. For those with experience in the food industry, maybe they are already knowledgeable, but you would need to prove this rather than assume it is true. It would be up to you to determine what additional training they would need.

For new employees, "On-the-job" training (OJT) is very effective once they have learned some basics in why food safety is important. Even long-time employees may benefit from more training if you feel they are not demonstrating food safety habits that meet the current standards in the food code. An OJT coach or supervisor can demonstrate the skills that are needed to prepare food safely and broaden their understanding of food safety. It's best to organize the training so that each task that the employee is responsible for is covered. For all employees, new and existing, there are numerous training resources on-line. On-line materials are particularly helpful as they often come in many languages. In addition, there are videos and DVDs that you can purchase or even "rent" or borrow from your local restaurant association. Another way that we conduct training is to do voluntary food safety inspections or what is also known as third party audits. Once classroom and on-the-job training are complete, these inspections will highlight not only areas in need of improvement but sometimes reveal practices that are hazardous. This also gives us the opportunity to demonstrate to the employees proper ways to prepare food safely if unsafe practices are observed.

Whatever method or combination of methods you use, it is important to keep on top of the training and make sure that it is ongoing and not a one time event. You do have many responsibilities and food safety is just one of them. But, if ignored, the consequences are significant.

HACCP

HACCP (Hazard Analysis Critical Control Point) is a food safety program that systematically identifies, evaluates and controls food safety hazards. The Pillsbury Company developed HACCP for the National Aeronautics and Space administration (NASA) to provide the safest and highest quality food for the astronauts in the space program. Because of its success, it was adopted by the meat, poultry and seafood industries in the 1990's and by the juice industry in 2002. To simplify this, take a look at the HA part of HACCP. This is the "hazard analysis" which is simply identifying hazards (biological, chemical or physical) that are likely to cause illness or injury if not controlled. Then, take a look at the CCP part of HACCP. This is the "critical control point" or the "essential step or steps" we can take to prevent, eliminate or reduce the hazards identified. The critical control points are the points in food handling processes where a loss of control may result in an unacceptable health risk. Critical control points are usually control measures such as cooking, cooling or refrigerating potentially hazardous foods (time/temperature control for safety foods).

So, let's use what we've learned so far using the example of preparing and cooking a whole turkey. If we were to conduct a "hazard analysis", we would most likely identify salmonella as the most obvious hazard (a biological hazard) that could cause illness. Now, for the "critical control point" (or what we call the "essential step") we must identify a step to prevent, eliminate or reduce the hazard. In this case, cooking the turkey thoroughly would be the "critical control point" as this would reduce the salmonella to safe levels. Not cooking the turkey will lead to an unacceptable health risk. That is the gist of a HACCP plan.

The Food Code clearly establishes that the implementation of HACCP at retail should be a voluntary effort. If, however, you plan on conducting certain specialized processes that carry considerably higher risk, you should consult your regulatory authority to see if you are required to have a HACCP plan. Examples of specialized processes include:
1. Smoking food for food preservation rather than as a method of flavor enhancement;
2. Curing food;
3. Using food additives or adding components such as vinegar for food preservation rather than as a method of flavor enhancement or to render a food not potentially hazardous (time/temperature control of food safety);
4. Packaging food using reduced oxygen packaging (ROP);
5. Operating a molluscan shellfish life-support system display tank used to store and display shellfish that are offered for human consumption;
6. Sprouting seeds or beans; or
7. Custom processing animals that are for personal use as food and not for sale or service in a food establishment.

Even if you don't plan on conducting one of these specialized processes, you still need to know what HACCP is all about. The description above is a very simplistic picture of what HACCP is about, but there is a lot more to it than that. There are technically seven HACCP principles as shown in the steps below.

HACCP PRINCIPLE #1 - CONDUCTING A HAZARD ANALYSIS

The first principle is conducting a hazard analysis. Again, conducting a hazard analysis is simply identifying hazards (biological, chemical or physical) that are likely to cause illness or injury if not controlled.

HACCP PRINCIPLE #2 - DETERMINING THE CRITICAL CONTROL POINTS (CCPs)

The second principle is identifying the critical control points (CCPs) that are necessary to prevent, eliminate or reduce the hazard. The critical control points are the points in food handling processes where a loss of control may result in an unacceptable health risk. Critical control points are usually control measures such as cooking, cooling or refrigerating potentially hazardous (time/temperature control for safety foods).

HACCP PRINCIPLE #3 - ESTABLISH CRITICAL LIMITS (CLs)

The third principle is establishing the Critical Limits (CLs). A critical limit is a numeric value, usually a maximum or a minimum value, that is required to prevent, eliminate or reduce the hazard identified in the hazard analysis. Critical limits are usually derived from regulatory standards such as required cooking temperatures.

HACCP PRINCIPLE # 4- ESTABLISH MONITORING PROCEDURES

The fourth principle is establishing the monitoring procedures. Monitoring is the act of observing and making measurements to determine if critical limits are being met.

HACCP PRINCIPLE # 5- ESTABLISH CORRECTIVE ACTIONS

The fifth principle is establishing corrective actions. These are actions that must be taken if our critical limits are not met. The operator decides what the actions will be, communicates those actions to the employees, and trains them in making the right decisions. This preventive approach is the heart of a HACCP plan.

HACCP PRINCIPLE #6 - ESTABLISH VERIFICATION PROCEDURES

The sixth principle is verifying that the system is operating according to the plan. More specifically, this principle is about making sure that the system is scientifically-sound to effectively control the hazards. In addition, this step ensures that the system is operating according to what is specified in the plan. Designated individuals, like the manager, periodically make observations of employees' monitoring activities, calibrate equipment and temperature measuring devices, review records/actions, and discuss procedures with the employees. All of these activities are for the purpose of ensuring that the HACCP plan is addressing the food safety concerns and, if not, checking to see where it needs to be modified or improved.

HACCP PRINCIPLE #7 - ESTABLISH RECORD KEEPING PROCEDURES

There are certain written records or kinds of documentation that are needed in order to verify that the system is working. These records will normally involve the HACCP plan itself and any monitoring, corrective actions, or calibration records produced in the operation of a the HACCP system. Verification records may also be included. Records maintained in a HACCP system serve to document that an ongoing, effective system is in place. Record keeping should be as simple as possible in order to make it more likely that employees will have the time to keep the records.

Now, let's get back to our HACCP plan for the turkey. We already determined that the main hazard associated with turkey is salmonella (which is a biological hazard) and that the critical control point or "essential step" we can take to prevent, eliminate or reduce the salmonella is to cook the turkey thoroughly. The remaining 5 principles build on those first two. The table below describes the 7 principles involved with HACCP based on this simple turkey example.

HACCP Principles Applied to Cooking a Raw Turkey

HACCP Principle	Turkey HACCP
1. Conducting a Hazard Analysis (HA) - This is identifying hazards (biological, chemical, or physical) that are most likely to occur.	Salmonella (biological hazard)
2. Establishing Critical Control Points (CCP) - This is determining the "essential step or steps" that must be taken to prevent, eliminate or reduce the hazard.	Cooking - this will reduce the salmonella to safe levels. Not cooking the turkey thoroughly will lead to an unacceptable risk.
3. Establishing Critical Limits (CL) - This is determining the critical limit (which is a numeric value, usually a maximum or a minimum value), which is required to prevent, eliminate or reduce the hazard identified in the hazard analysis.	165 degrees for 15 seconds is the minimal internal cooking temperature to reduce the salmonella to safe levels.
4. Monitoring Procedures - These are procedures taken to assure that we are meeting our critical limit.	Checking the internal temperature of the turkey with a thermometer.
5. Corrective Actions - These are actions to be taken if our critical limit is not met.	If the turkey has not been cooked to 165 degrees, continue cooking the turkey until it has reached 165 degrees for 15 seconds.
6. Verification - This is making sure that the plan is working and being followed by employees. This may include making sure that the critical limits are being met, that records are being maintained and accurate, or that monitoring equipment is working properly.	Reviewing temperature logs on a regular basis to make sure all turkeys have been cooked to 165 degrees, making sure logs are kept on file, or calibrating thermometers that are used to check the cooking temperatures of the turkey.
7. Record Keeping - This is keeping written records, such as temperature logs, that document that critical limits are being met. These records may include logs for calibrating the thermometer, or even logs documenting any corrective actions.	Documenting cooking temperatures for the turkey on temperature logs. You may want to document that thermometers have been calibrated on a calibration logs. You may even want to have verification logs that document that employees have checked temperatures properly.

In order for any HACCP plan to be effective, a strong foundation of procedures that address the basic operations and sanitation conditions within an operation must first be developed and implemented. These "foundation of procedures" are usually called "prerequisite programs". These prerequisite programs can include training programs for your managers and employees, having a pest control program, having buyer specifications, or any other standard operating procedures you may have developed, from cleaning and sanitizing to washing hands.

This is a very simple example of HACCP for an individual item that one might have in a restaurant. Obviously, if you were to have a 7 step HACCP plan for every menu item or food type, the HACCP plan would be overwhelming and therefore ineffective.

A more practical type of HACCP plan for the restaurant industry focuses on the types of processes (or food preparation procedures) that are commonly used in this industry. This is referred to as the "process approach" to HACCP. This is a HACCP plan that, rather than focusing on individual food items, will focus on types of food processes. Most food processes can be classified into three types: process 1 - foods that are prepared and require no cooking at the retail level; process 2 - foods that are prepared for same day service and require cooking and sometimes holding; and process 3 - foods that involve complex food preparation such as preparing, cooking, cooling, reheating, and holding.

These three types of processes are also defined by how many times the food goes through the danger zone. With process 1, the food may at some point be in the danger zone, but will not pass all the way through the danger zone. This is the "No Cook" process. Examples of this would be raw ready-to-eat foods such as sushi, sashimi, or raw oysters. This may also include salads or sandwiches containing deli meat and cheese or foods that require no cooking or preparation such as yogurt.

With process 2, the food will only go through the danger zone once and is classified as "Same Day Service". Examples of this type of process would be foods that would be cooked and held hot until served (or cooked and served immediately) such as fried chicken, hamburgers and French fries, or scrambled eggs.

Finally, with process 3, foods go through the danger zone more than once and are classified as "Complex" food preparation. Chicken salad would be a great example here. The chicken is received cold, is then cooked, is cooled; then prepared (cut and mixed with other ingredients) for the salad. The chicken has gone through the danger zone twice. Some items may go through the danger zone three times such as chili or stews in which the food is cooked, held, cooled, re-heated and held again.

As you can see, once the menu items are classified into one of these specific food preparation categories, managerial controls can be placed on each type of grouping to control the hazards.

Ultimately, the goal in applying HACCP principles in retail and food service is to have you, the operator, take purposeful actions to ensure safe food. You and your regulatory authority have a common objective in mind, providing safe, quality food to consumers. Your health inspector can help you achieve this common objective, but remember that the ultimate responsibility for food safety at the retail level lies with you and your ability to develop and maintain an effective food safety management system.

Complete Trips Through the Danger Zone

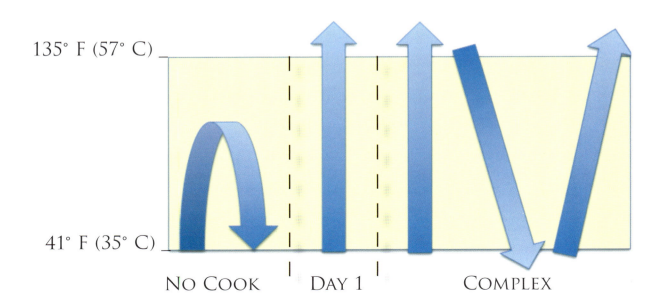

Chapter 9 - Quiz

1. The term "Active Managerial Control" refers to the industries' responsibility for developing and implementing a food safety program. These responsibilities do not include:
    A. Making sure that all employees have health insurance.
    B. Demonstrating knowledge in food safety.
    C. Prohibiting bare hand contact with ready-to-eat foods.
    D. Having a consumer advisory.

2. A training gap refers to the gap between:
    A. What all new employees know versus what the existing employees know.
    B. The gap between what an employee learned at their last job and what they have learned at their current job.
    C. The gap between what an employee knows and what they are required to know to do their job safely.
    D. All of the above

3. Job skills learned while working with a training coach is referred to as:
    A. A training gap.
    B. Classroom style training.
    C. On the job training.
    D. Distance learning.

4. A HACCP plan is only required when an establishment performs specialized processes, such as:
    A. Serving scrambled eggs to highly susceptible populations.
    B. Serving raw hamburgers to college students.
    C. Using a two bay sink for manual warewashing.
    D. Sprouting of seeds or beans.

5. According to the seven principles of HACCP, which of the following is an example of monitoring?
    A. Cooking the turkey thoroughly.
    B. Checking the temperature of the turkey with a calibrated bi-metalic stem thermometer.
    C. Writing down the temperature on the temperature log.
    D. Reviewing the temperature logs at the end of each month.

6. When cooking a turkey to reduce the salmonella to safe levels, the critical limit is:
    A. Cooking the turkey thoroughly.
    B. 165 degrees for 15 seconds.
    C. Making sure that the turkey has been cooked for 2 hours.
    D. Making sure the oven has been set to 350 degrees before placing the turkey in the oven.

Answer Key
1. A   2. C   3. C   4. D   5. B   6. B

Food Safety Acronyms

ANSI	American National Standards Institute
ASP	Amnesic Shellfish Poisoning
CCP	Critical Control Point
CDC	Center for Disease Control and Prevention
CFP	Conference of Food Protection
CL	Critical Limit
CFR	Code of Federal Regulation
EPA	Environmental Protection Agency
EPH	Environmental and Public Health
FATTOM	Food, Acidity, Temperature, Time, Oxygen, Moisture
FDA	Food and Drug Administration
FIFO	First-In / First-Out
FSIS	Food Safety Inspectional Services
GAP	Good Agricultural Practices
GMP	Good Manufacturing Practices
HACCP	Hazard Analysis Critical Control Point
IPM	Integrated Pest Management
MAP	Medical Atmosphere Packaging
MSDS	Material Safety Data Sheet
NASA	National Aeronautics and Space Administration
NSF	National Sanitation Foundation
NSP	Neurotoxic Shellfish Poisoning
OJT	On-the-Job-Training
OSHA	Occupational Safety and Health Administration
PCO	Pest Control Operator
PHF	Potentially Hazardous Foods
PIC	Person in Charge
PPE	Personal Protective Equipment
PPM	Parts per Million
PSP	Paralytic Shellfish Poisoning
ROP	Reduced Oxygen Packaging
RTE	Ready-to-Eat
SOP	Standard Operating Procedure
TCS	Time Temperature Control Safety
TTI	Time-Temperature Indicator
UHT	Ultra High Temperature
UL	Underwriters Laboratories
USDA	U.S Department of Agriculture

Index

Symbols

4 hour rule 12

A

abrasive cleaning 47, 48
acidic cleaning 47, 51
acidity 11
allergies 4, 19, 20, 25, 35, 37
aluminum 18

B

bacteria 1, 10, 11, 12, 13, 14, 15, 16, 17, 20, 24, 25, 29, 30, 34, 36, 38, 40, 41, 42, 45
bare hand contact 24, 25, 28, 64, 69
bimetal 31, 32
biological hazards 10
blast chiller 41
boiling point method 33

C

calibrating 32
carpeting 57, 62
CDC (Centers for Disease Control and Prevention) 3, 5, 56, 62
ceilings 57
cheese 14, 17, 18
chemical concentrations 48
chemical hazards 10, 18, 22
chlorine 48, 51
cleaning 44, 47, 50, 55, 56, 59, 62
cleaning agents 47
cockroaches 53
cold storage 34
consumer advisory 39
cooking 29, 38, 39, 42, 44, 68, 69
cooking temperatures 39
cooling 29, 40, 42
copper 18
cough 23
coving 57
Critical Control Points 4, 68

cross contamination 4, 30, 44
curing food 38, 66
cuts 14, 24, 29, 35
cutting boards 29, 30, 45, 47, 49, 58

D

day care centers 37
de-greasers 47
demonstrate knowledge 5
detergents 47
diarrhea 13, 14, 15, 16, 17, 19, 26, 28
dry storage 35

E

eggs 4, 8, 9, 22, 25, 30, 33, 37, 38, 39, 40, 44, 45, 49, 69
equipment & utensils 57, 58
Escherichia coli 26

F

facility design 57, 61
FAT TOM 10, 12, 13
FDA (Food and Drug Administration) 2, 3, 4, 5, 11, 38, 56, 58, 60, 61, 62, 63, 64
fever 13, 14, 15, 16, 26
fingernails 24
floors 51, 57
foodborne illness 1, 2, 3, 4, 5, 6, 7, 8, 9, 10, 14, 15, 18, 23, 26, 28, 33, 36, 39, 40, 43, 64
food code 2, 3
food contact surfaces 23, 48, 49, 51, 53, 58
food employee 5
freezer 21, 35, 36, 42, 45, 71
FSIS (Food Safety and Inspection Service) 3, 5
fungi 17, 18

G

galvanized 18
garbage 57, 60
gloves 7, 14, 20, 21, 22, 24, 25, 28, 30

H

HACCP (Hazard Analysis Critical Control Points) 4, 12, 36, 37, 38, 64, 66, 67, 68, 69
handwashing 4, 23, 24, 57, 58, 62
handwashing stations 57, 58
heat treated plant foods 8
hepatitis 15, 21, 26, 28
highly susceptible populations 8, 39, 43, 69
high risk populations 37
holding 29, 41, 42
hot water 24, 28, 43, 47, 48, 49, 58

I

ice 38, 43
ice point method 32, 33, 44
illness policy 23, 26, 43, 64
improper cleaning and sanitizing 7
internal temperature 31, 42, 43, 44, 45, 68
iodine 48, 51
IPM (integrated pest management) 53, 54, 55, 56

J

jaundice 15, 26
jewelry 18, 24

K

L

laser 31
latex 20, 25
lead 13, 18, 36, 66, 68
lighting 57, 60, 61

M

maintenance 57, 62
major food allergens 4, 19
manual warewashing 47
master cleaning schedule 47, 50
melons 9, 37, 73
mice 53
microwave cooking 39
milk 9, 13, 14, 16, 31, 34, 37, 44, 45
moisture 12, 39
molds 10, 17, 18, 34
monitoring temperatures 29, 30

N

non-absorbent 57
non-food contact surfaces 58
norovirus 15, 21, 26
nursing homes 37
nuts 19, 22

O

outbreak 2
oxygen 12, 38, 66

P

parasites 10, 15, 33
parts per million 48
pasteurized eggs 37
pathogenic microorganisms 10
PCO (pest control operator) 53, 54, 55, 56
personal hygiene 4, 7, 10, 15, 21, 23, 26, 29, 36, 42, 58, 61, 65
pests 53, 54, 55
pewter 18
PHF's (potentially hazardous foods) 8, 12, 30, 33, 35-42
physical hazards 10, 18, 22
PIC (person in charge) 3, 4, 5, 6, 23, 26, 28, 45, 64
plan review 57, 61
plumbing 57, 59
poor personal hygiene 7, 23, 36
potentially hazardous food 4
PPM (parts per million) 48
preparation 29, 35, 36
produce 37
purchase & receiving 33

Q

quaternary ammonium compounds 48
quats 48, 51

R

rats 53
raw foods 25, 30
raw oysters 39
reduced oxygen packaging 38, 66
refrigerator 7, 12, 13, 14, 35, 36, 41, 44, 45, 51, 58, 71
refuse 57, 60, 75

reheating 29, 41, 42
reputable vendor 33
reputable vendors 7, 16, 17, 54
restroom 24, 25, 28, 57
roasts 41
RTE (Ready to eat Foods) 4, 7, 13, 24, 25, 28, 30, 33, 35, 39, 40, 43, 44, 49, 69

S

salads containing PHF/TCS foods 37
salmonella 14, 26, 68
sanitizing 4, 6, 7, 18, 44, 47, 48, 49, 50, 51, 64, 68, 77
service & display 43
sewer 57, 59
shellfish 8, 14, 15, 16, 19, 22, 30, 33, 38, 39, 44, 66
shigella 14, 26
sneeze 23, 43, 46
sores 24
sore throat 26
spoilage organisms 10, 17
storage 29, 34, 35
symptoms 13, 15, 16, 17, 19

T

TCS (time/temperature control for safety) 8, 12, 30, 33, 35-42
temperature danger zone 11, 12, 20, 30, 36, 40, 41, 42
thawing 36, 45
thermistor 32
thermocouple 32
thermometers 30, 31, 32, 43, 68
three bay sink 47, 48, 50, 52, 63
time and temperature abuse 7
time as a public health control 36, 42, 46
time temperature abuse 36
time/temperature control for safety food 4
time/temperature indicator 32
toxins 10, 12, 16, 18, 22, 40

U

under-cooked 39
uniform 24, 25
USDA (United States Department of Agriculture) 3, 5, 34, 56, 62

utensils 4, 7, 10, 14, 18, 25, 26, 30, 43, 46, 47, 49, 50, 51, 58

V

variance 38, 76
vegetables 8, 10, 11, 13, 14, 16, 37, 40, 72, 74
ventilation 51, 57, 60
ventilation hoods 51
virus 1, 10, 14–22, 15, 25
vomiting 13, 14, 15, 16, 17, 21, 26, 28

W

walls 57
warewashing machines 47
wash hands 24
wedding band 24

X

Y

yeasts 10, 17, 18

Z